The Principles of Endodontics

D0814797

NSCC-INSTITUTE OF TECHNOLOGY
LIBRARY
DISCARD
5685 LEEDS STREET
HALIFAX, NOVA SCOTIA   B3K 2T3

ACADIA UNIVERSITY LIBRARY
Library
Acadia Street
WOLFVILLE, NOVA SCOTIA, CANADA

The Principles of Endodontics

SECOND EDITION

Edited by

Shanon Patel

Justin J. Barnes

NSCC-INSTITUTE OF TECHNOLOGY
LIBRARY
5685 LEEDS STREET
HALIFAX, NOVA SCOTIA   B3K 2T3

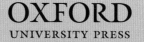
OXFORD
UNIVERSITY PRESS

Great Clarendon Street, Oxford OX2 6DP,
United Kingdom

Oxford University Press is a department of the University of Oxford.
It furthers the University's objective of excellence in research, scholarship,
and education by publishing worldwide. Oxford is a registered trade mark of
Oxford University Press in the UK and in certain other countries

© Oxford University Press, 2013

The moral rights of the authors have been asserted

First Edition published 2005
Second Edition published 2013

Impression: 1

All rights reserved. No part of this publication may be reproduced,
stored in a retrieval system, or transmitted, in any form or by any means,
without the prior permission in writing of Oxford University Press,
or as expressly permitted by law, by licence or under terms agreed with the appropriate
reprographics rights organization. Enquiries concerning reproduction
outside the scope of the above should be sent to the Rights Department,
Oxford University Press, at the address above

You must not circulate this work in any other form
and you must impose the same condition on any acquirer

British Library Cataloguing in Publication Data

Data available

ISBN 978-0-19-965751-3

Printed and bound by
Bell & Bain Ltd, Glasgow

Oxford University Press makes no representation, express or implied,
that the drug dosages in this book are correct. Readers must therefore always
check the product information and clinical procedures with the most up-to-date
published product information and data sheets provided by the manufacturers and
the most recent codes of conduct and safety regulations. The authors and the publishers
do not accept responsibility or legal liability for any errors in the text or for the misuse
or misapplication of material in this work. Except where otherwise stated, drug dosages
and recommendations are for the non-pregnant adult who is not breast-feeding.

Links to third party websites are provided by Oxford in good faith and
for information only. Oxford disclaims any responsibillty for the materials
contained in any third party website referenced in this work.

Dedication

This book is dedicated to:

Almas, Genie and Zarina
Shanon Patel

Kathleen and Michael
Justin J. Barnes

Foreword

Endodontology is a core subject for the undergraduate dental student, providing both technical and intellectual challenges. It could be argued that molar root canal treatment is the most demanding of practical exercises a general dental practitioner will face, combining as it does diagnostic and treatment planning skills and precise technical procedures. Thus, a strong foundation in this subject is pivotal to continuing high quality provision of dental care throughout the professional career of the graduate. Endodontology has been the Cinderella of the restorative dental specialties and, with the advent of implants, the importance of endodontics as a treatment option has been diminished. The continuing development of the broad science of endodontology including microbiology, immunology and dental materials science ensures that the arguments in favour of preservation of teeth with pulpal and periradicular disease are understood fully and can be rightly and confidently included in holistic treatment planning of patients.

This textbook provides an excellent foundation for understanding the principles of endodontology, and specifically the practice of root canal treatment and subsequent restoration of the root filled tooth. Students, at whatever level, benefit from clear guidelines based upon previous and current scientific investigation, illustrative material that shows the reader what can be done and the level to which they should aspire. This book is written by specialist endodontists at the top of their game. The quality of the clinical cases is inspirational and the clear text and accompanying diagrams provide the key information that both undergraduates and general dental practitioners require to develop and improve their skills.

Training to be a specialist takes time and huge commitment and the knowledge and experience accumulated over the years may be unselfishly passed on to others. The authors of this book have made this obligation and the reader will be inspired to do better for their patients.

Professor William P Saunders
BDS, DSc (hc), PhD, FDS RCS Edin, FDS RCPS Glas, FDS RCS Eng, MRD, FHEA, FCDSHK
Professor of Endodontology / Honorary Consultant in Restorative Dentistry
University of Dundee

Preface to the second edition

The aim of this second edition is to provide a contemporary comprehensive guide to endodontics. This edition covers the many advances in endodontic knowledge, techniques, materials, and equipment since the first edition was published. The intended readership remains undergraduate dental students who wish to develop an understanding of 'why' and 'how' safe, predictable, and effective endodontic treatment is carried out. The book will also benefit recent graduates who want to refresh their knowledge and the established clinicians who are continuing their professional development.

The style of the new edition remains simple and user-friendly. There are several changes since the first edition. Existing chapters have been significantly revised and updated. We have enlisted a group of respected academics, and also up-and-coming endodontists to help us with this project. In the first edition, there were distinct sections on theory and practice of endodontics. This has been revised for ease of reference; applicable chapters cover essential theory and this is followed by a guide to the practice of endodontics. New chapters include restoration of the endodontically treated tooth and dento-legal aspects to endodontics. There has been an effort to use the most up-to-date terminology in endodontics and ensure consistency of terminology throughout the book. References are kept to a minimum with readers being invited to explore suggested further reading at the end of each chapter.

We hope that this second edition will continue to help your understanding of the principles of endodontics so that you can achieve satisfying results and goals in your clinical practice.

Shanon Patel
Justin J. Barnes

Acknowledgements

The editors would like to express their gratitude to Michael Manogue and Richard Walker who were instrumental in developing the first edition of this novel book.

We would like to thank all the contributors for sparing their valuable time.

We would like to acknowledge our colleagues and other publishers who kindly gave permission to reproduce their superb illustrative material.

We express thanks to the staff at Oxford University Press, especially Geraldine Jeffers, Senior Commissioning Editor, for their advice, encouragement, and patience.

Finally, we are indebted to our families and friends who have been pillars of support throughout this process.

Figures 2.2, 2.5, 2.6, 2.10 Courtesy of Drs Hélio Lopes and José Siqueira.

Figures 2.8, 2.14, 2.15 Courtesy Dr Domenico Ricucci.

Figure 2.18 Courtesy of Drs Ricardo C Fraga and Flávio F Alves.

Figures 2.19, 2.22 Adapted from Siqueira J and Rôças I (2011) Case 1.1 Microbiology of primary periapical periodontitis. In: Patel S and Duncan H (eds) *Pitt Ford's Problem-Based Learning in Endodontology*, with permission from Wiley-Blackwell.

Figure 4.2 Adapted from Nair PNR, Duncan HF, Pitt Ford TR, Luder HU (2008) Histological, ultrastructural and quantitative investigations on the response of healthy human pulps to experimental capping with mineral trioxide aggregate: a randomized controlled trial. *International Endodontic Journal* **41**: 128–50. Printed with permission from Wiley-Blackwell.

Figure 4.3 Courtesy of Drs Conor Durack and Edward Brady.

Figures 4.7, 4.8, 7.3, 7.27 Adapted from Patel and Duncan (2011) *Pitt Ford's Problem-Based Learning in Endodontology*. Printed with permission from Wiley-Blackwell.

Figure 5.59 Courtesy of Dr Bhavin Bhuva.

Figure 6.13 Courtesy of Dr Arthur Greenwood.

Figure 6.46 Courtesy of Mrs Heather Pitt Ford.

Figures 7.1, 7.2, 7.4, 7.5, 7.6, 7.8, 7.19, 7.24 Courtesy of Dr Pareet Shah.

Figures 7.15, 7.20, 7.21, 7.22 Adapted from Mannocci, Cavalli and Gagliani (2008) *Adhesive Restoration of Endodontically Treated Teeth*. Printed with permission from Quintessence Publishing.

Figure 7.23 Courtesy of Dr Edward Sammut.

Figure 8.9 Adapted from Patel S, Wilson R, Foschi F, Dawood A, Mannocci F (2012) The detection of periapical pathology using digital periapical radiography and cone beam computed tomography – part 2–1 year post treatment outcome. *International Endodontic Journal* **45**, 711–23. Printed with permission from Wily-Blackwell.

Figure 9.7 Courtesy of Dr Tan Boon Tik.

Figure 9.19 Courtesy of Dr Tom Bereznicki.

Table 10.1 and Figures 10.1, 10.7 Courtesy of Dr Len D'Cruz, personal communication.

Figure 10.6 Courtesy of Dr Steve Williams. Adapted from Patel and Duncan (2011) *Pitt Ford's Problem-Based Learning in Endodontology*. Printed with permission from Wiley-Blackwell.

Contents

About the editors

Shanon Patel BDS, MSc, MClinDent, MFDS RCS (Eng), MRD RCS (Edin), PhD

Shanon divides his time between working in specialist practice in central London, and teaching future specialist endodontists in the Endodontic Postgraduate Unit at King's College London. Shanon's PhD thesis assessed the applications of cone beam computed tomography in Endodontics.

He has published over 45 papers in peer reviewed scientific journals, and also co-edited two undergraduate textbooks *The Principles of Endodontics* (Oxford University Press) and *Pitt Ford's Problem-Based Learning in Endodontology* (Wiley–Blackwell). He is frequently asked to lecture nationally and internationally on all aspects of endodontics. He has also served on the council of the British Endodontic Society.

Justin J. Barnes BSc, BDS, MFDS RCPS (Glasg), MClinDent, MRD RCS (Edin)

Justin studied anatomy and dentistry at Queen's University Belfast, graduating in 2004. He worked in general dental practice for one year as a vocational dental practitioner. He then worked for two years as a senior house officer in oral and maxillofacial surgery and restorative dentistry at the Royal Victoria Hospital, Belfast. Justin has also worked in the emergency dental services. Justin completed his specialist training in endodontology at King's College London Dental Institute in 2010.

Justin offers a specialist endodontic service in Northern Ireland. He also teaches undergraduate dental students at the Centre for Dental Education, Queen's University Belfast. Justin has published several papers in peer reviewed journals and he delivers endodontic educational courses for dentists.

About the contributors

Avijit Banerjee BDS, MSc, PhD (Lond), FDS (Rest Dent), FDS RCS (Eng), FHEA

Specialist in Prosthodontics, Periodontics and Restorative Dentistry
Professor of Cariology & Operative Dentistry/Honorary Consultant in Restorative Dentistry,
Department of Conservative Dentistry,
King's College London Dental Institute, London, UK

Justin J. Barnes BSc, BDS, MFDS RCPS (Glasg), MClinDent, MRD RCS (Edin)

Specialist in Endodontics, Northern Ireland
Centre for Dental Education, Queen's University Belfast, UK

Bhavin Bhuva BDS, MFDS RCS (Eng), MClinDent, MRD RCS (Edin)

Specialist in Endodontics, Hertfordshire, Essex, and London, UK
Consultant in Endodontics,
Department of Restorative Dentistry and Traumatology,
King's College Hospital, London, UK

Edward Brady BChD, MJDF RCS (Eng), MClinDent, M Endo RCS (Edin)

Specialist in Endodontics
Postgraduate Endodontic Unit,
King's College London Dental Institute, London, UK

Bun San Chong BDS, MSc, PhD (Lond); LDS, FDS RCS (Eng); MFGDP (UK); MRD, FHEA

Specialist in Endodontics
Professor of Restorative Dentistry/Honorary Consultant,
Institute of Dentistry, Barts and The London School of Medicine and Dentistry, Queen Mary,
University of London, London, UK

Len D'Cruz BDS, LDS RCS (Eng), Dip FOd, MFGDP (UK), LLM, PgCert Med Ed

General dental practitioner, London, UK
Dento-legal advisor, Dental Protection Limited, London, UK

Conor Durack BDS NUI, MFDS RCSI, MClinDent, M Endo RCS (Edin)

Specialist in Endodontics
Postgraduate Endodontic Unit,
King's College London Dental Institute, London, UK

Shalini Kanagasingam BDS, MFDS RCS (Eng), MClinDent, MRD RCS (Edin)

Lecturer and Endodontist
Department of Operative Dentistry, Faculty of Dentistry,
Universiti Kebangsaan Malaysia, Kuala Lumpur, Malaysia

Francesco Mannocci MD, DDS, PhD

Specialist in Endodontics and Restorative Dentistry
Professor, and Head of Endodontology/Honorary Consultant,
Postgraduate Endodontic Unit,
King's College London Dental Institute, London, UK

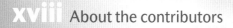

Shanon Patel BDS, MSc, MClinDent, MFDS RCS (Eng), MRD RCS (Edin), PhD

Specialist in Endodontics
Postgraduate Endodontic Unit,
King's College London Dental Institute, London, UK

Isabela N. Rôças DDS, MSc, PhD

Adjunct Professor, Department of Endodontics, and Head, Molecular Microbiology Laboratory,
Faculty of Dentistry,
Estácio de Sá University, Rio de Janeiro, RJ, Brazil

José F. Siqueira Jr DDS, MSc, PhD

Professor and Chairman, Department of Endodontics and Molecular Microbiology Laboratory,
Faculty of Dentistry,
Estácio de Sá University, Rio de Janeiro, RJ, Brazil

Abbreviations

BMPs	Bone morphogenic proteins
CBCT	Cone beam computed tomography
CCD	Charge-coupled devices
CEJ	Cemento–enamel junction
CMOS	Complementary metal oxide semiconductors
EAL	Electronic apex locator
EBV	Epstein–Barr virus
EDJ	Enamel–dentine junction
EDTA	Ethylenediaminetetracetic acid
GIC	Glass ionomer cement
GP	Gutta-percha
HCMV	Human cytomegalovirus
IGF	Insulin-like growth factor
IRM	Intermediate Restorative Material
ISO	International Organization for Standardization
MAF	master apical file
MI	Minimally invasive
MTA	Mineral Trioxide Aggregate
NaOCl	Sodium hypochlorite
NiTi	Nickel-titanium
NSAID	Non-steroidal anti-inflammatory drugs
PDGF	Platelet-derived growth factor
PMNs	Polymorphonuclear neutrophils
PUI	Passive ultrasonic irrigation
TGF	Transforming growth factor

1
Introduction

Shanon Patel and Justin J. Barnes

Chapter contents

What is endodontics?

Endodontics literally means the science of the inside of the tooth. The term has its origins from the Greek 'endo' meaning 'within' and 'odont' meaning 'tooth'. The suffix '-ics' means 'area of work and study'.

Teeth and their supporting tissues may become involved in dental infections that are caused by microbes from the oral microflora. These microbes, primarily bacteria, may cause disease around teeth (periodontal disease) and/or inside teeth (endodontic disease).

Endodontic disease affects the enamel, dentine, pulp, and periapical tissues. They are characterized by loss of the integrity of the enamel and dentine; in advanced cases the pulp may also become (in)directly involved. Examples include dental caries (Fig. 1.1), dental trauma (Fig. 1.2), tooth surface loss (Fig. 1.3a,b) which may result in irreversible pulpitis, and ultimately periapical periodontitis (Fig. 1.4).

Endodontology is the branch of dental science concerned with the form, function, health, injuries to, and diseases of, the dentine, dental pulp, and the adjacent periapical tissues.

Endodontics is the branch of clinical dentistry concerned with the prevention, diagnosis, and treatment of endodontic disease. Essentially, endodontics involves all procedures required for the maintenance of healthy teeth and, where teeth have become diseased, treatments required to return teeth to a healthy status. Understanding endodontics requires knowledge of the biological processes affecting teeth and their supporting tissue (Chapter 2), and knowledge of the related basic science subjects, including:

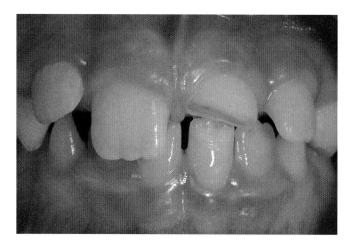

Figure 1.2 Dental trauma: complicated crown fracture of a maxillary central incisor tooth. There has been a fracture involving enamel and dentine, and the pulp has been exposed.

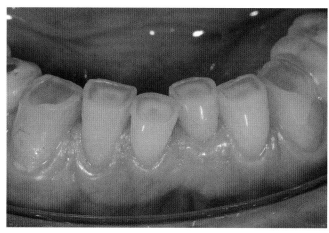

(a)

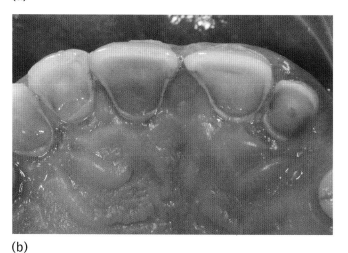

(b)

Figure 1.3 Tooth surface loss: (a) attrition and erosion affecting the mandibular anterior teeth and (b) erosion, nearing pulpal exposures, affecting the palatal surfaces of the maxillary anterior teeth.

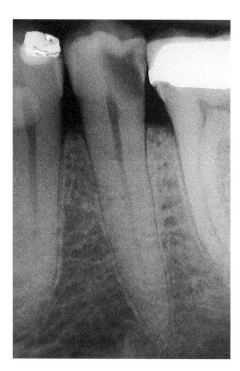

Figure 1.1 Dental caries associated with a mandibular premolar tooth.

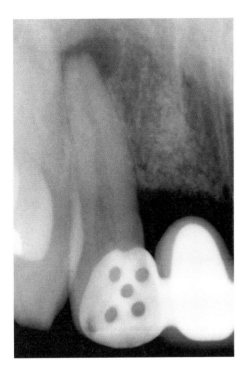

Figure 1.4 Periapical periodontitis associated with a maxillary incisor tooth.

- **Embryology**, in particular, the development of teeth and their supporting tissues;
- **Anatomy**, in particular, the structures of teeth and their supporting tissues;
- **Histology**, in particular, the microscopic structures of enamel, dentine and pulp;
- **Physiology**, in particular, the normal functions of the pulp;
- **Pathology**, in particular, the cause and effects of disease of the pulp and periapical tissues;
- **Microbiology**, in particular, oral microbes and infections;
- **Pharmacology**, in particular, drugs used in general dentistry and endodontics;
- **Dental materials science**, in particular, the instruments and materials used in endodontics.

Which clinical conditions require endodontic management?

Patients with endodontic disease may present in a variety of ways. One patient may be suffering from severe orofacial pain and swelling; whilst another patient may be completely symptom-free. The clinical conditions that may require endodontic treatment are:

- Dental caries (Fig. 1.1)
- Traumatized teeth (Fig. 1.2)
- Tooth surface loss (Fig. 1.3a,b)

- Cracked teeth
- Pulpitis
- Periapical periodontitis: acute, suppurative, and chronic (Fig. 1.4)
- Root resorption.

It is only with a thorough understanding of the subject that the clinician will be able to effectively examine the patient and arrive at a correct diagnosis (Chapter 3).

What are the aims and scope of endodontics?

The aim of endodontic treatment is to prevent or treat periapical periodontitis by controlling infection. Essential components to achieving this aim are:

- Disinfection of teeth. This ranges from removing caries-affected dentine (Chapter 4) to a thorough disinfecting of the root canal system (Chapter 5).
- Sealing of teeth after root canal preparation to prevent reinfection. This ranges from placement of a root canal filling (Chapter 6) to providing a well-fitting definitive coronal restoration (Chapter 7).

It is important to appreciate that endodontics is not simply concerned with root canals and root canal treatment. The discipline plays a much wider role in the general dental care of patients. The scope of endodontics includes:

- Diagnosis of orofacial pain (Chapter 3)
- Pulp preservation therapies (Chapter 4)
- Root canal treatment (Chapters 5 and 6)
- Bleaching of endodontically treated teeth
- Restoration of endodontically treated teeth (Chapter 7)
- Advanced endodontic procedures: root canal retreatment and surgical endodontics (Chapter 9)
- Management of dental trauma.

What does it take to be competent?

All dentists should be able to carry out *safe* and *effective* endodontic treatment. You should only carry out treatment if you are sure that you are competent to do it. Competence is attained through sound theoretical knowledge together with adequate clinical experience and skills.

During your undergraduate dental training, it is imperative that:

- You attend teaching sessions and carry out self-directed learning;
- You gain experience using simulated and extracted teeth before embarking on treating patients;
- You reflect on your laboratory and clinical performance, and the feedback given by your supervisors. Reflections should be documented in a logbook.

After your undergraduate training, it is important that you continue to maintain your professional knowledge and competence. This can be achieved through private study, reading journals, and attending lectures and courses. Continuing professional development will allow you to keep up to date with modern trends. It is also important that you continue to reflect on your work as a qualified clinician. You need to be aware of your limitations and recognize when referral to a specialist is necessary for more advanced endodontic procedures (Chapter 9). You also need to recognize when things go wrong, how to manage these situations and prevent them from occurring again (Chapter 10).

Competency in endodontics requires the use of rubber dam (Fig. 1.5). It is of paramount importance that you continue to use rubber dam throughout your professional career. Rubber dam isolation is mandatory for all endodontic cases because it:

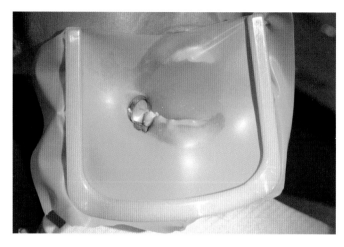

Figure 1.5 Rubber dam isolation during endodontic treatment.

- Prevents contamination of teeth by saliva;
- Protects the patient's oropharynx from instruments, debris, and disinfectants;
- Encourages the clinician to use acceptable disinfectants;
- Improves access and vision;
- Improves patient comfort;
- Increases clinician efficiency.

How has endodontics developed?

Endodontic disease and its management have been well chronicled. Ancient civilizations believed that toothache and dental disease was caused by a tooth worm. Historical management of endodontic disease has included primitive dental drills, herbal remedies, cauterizing the pulp, placement of arsenic into the root canal, and extraction.

It was not until the 19th century that microbes became associated with endodontic disease. Miller (1894)[1] was the first to demonstrate the presence of bacteria in samples retrieved from the pulp. Other developments in the 1800s included the invention of the reclining dental chair, introduction of the rubber dam, and discovery of X-rays.

The development of endodontics was hampered in the early 20th century by the theory that dental infection was a source for systemic disease (Focal Infection Theory). This led to extraction becoming the treatment of choice for endodontic disease. Since the 1950s, the Focal Infection Theory has largely been dispelled and there have been many developments in endodontics. Investigations in the 1960s confirmed that infection within the tooth is essential for periapical periodontitis to

occur. A classical study[2] revealed that when pulps were exposed to oral microbes, endodontic disease developed in normal rats; whilst, in germ-free rats, the pulps and periapical tissues remained healthy. The 1970s and 1980s increased our understanding of the microbiology of infected root canals; and the ways in which irrigants, agitation of irrigants, and medicaments can disinfect root canals.

Since the 1990s our knowledge of the nature of endodontic disease has significantly improved including microbial biofilms, the causes of post-treatment persistent disease, and the factors which influence the outcome of endodontic treatment. There have also been advancements in materials, equipment, and techniques including: cone beam computed tomography (CBCT), nickel-titanium (NiTi) files, newer generations of electronic apex locators, magnification devices, alternative bioactive root canal filling materials, and endodontic microsurgery. These developments have improved the diagnosis, consistency, safety, and efficiency in endodontics as well as improving patient comfort.

---

[1] Miller W (1894) An introduction in the study of the bacteriopathology of the dental pulp. *Dental Cosmos* **36**, 505.

[2] Kakehashi S, Stanley HR, Fitzgerald RJ (1965) The effects of surgical exposures of dental pulps in germ-free and conventional laboratory rats. *Oral Surgery, Oral Medicine, and Oral Pathology* **20**, 340–9.

So, what's in store for endodontics? Some clinicians and manufacturers claim that endodontics is on the decline and dental implants are a superior treatment option. For teeth that are already missing or have a hopeless prognosis, dental implants can be an excellent replacement option. Recent studies have shown that the survival rate of endodontically treated teeth is similar, if not better, than that of dental implants. Therefore, when possible, teeth should be saved! There are numerous advantages to preventing and treating endodontic disease so that teeth can be retained in a healthy state. These include: more cost-effective and expedient treatment and retention of the periodontal ligament.

The future of endodontics looks to be exciting with prospects of revascularization of root canals and the regeneration of the diseased pulp and dentine.

What is the purpose of this textbook?

The purpose of this textbook is to provide a contemporary comprehensive guide to endodontics. The intended readership is undergraduate dental students who wish to develop an understanding of 'why' and 'how' safe, predictable, and effective endodontics may be carried out. This book covers the essential theory of 'why' endodontic treatment is performed, and provides a step-by-step guide to the clinical practicalities of 'how' endodontic treatment is performed. Apart from being an adjunct to undergraduate dental teaching, this book acts as a refresher to recently qualified dentists and as an update to the established clinician who is continuing their professional development.

Summary points

- Endodontics is a branch of clinical dentistry concerned with the prevention, diagnosis, and treatment of diseases of the enamel, dentine, pulp, and periapical tissues. There are a wide range of clinical conditions which require endodontic management. The ultimate aim of endodontics is to prevent or treat periapical periodontitis.

- Endodontics involves the diagnosis of orofacial pain, pulp preservation therapies, root canal treatment, restoration of the endodontically-treated tooth, and advanced endodontic procedures such as root canal retreatment and surgical endodontics.

- You must be competent to carry out endodontic treatment. It is of paramount importance that you use rubber dam for all endodontic cases.

- Endodontics continues to develop and it is important that you keep up to date with these developments.

2

Life of a tooth

*José F. Siqueira Jr
and Isabela N. Rôças*

Chapter contents

Introduction

Dentine and pulp share the same embryologic origin and are intimately integrated in terms of anatomy and physiology; therefore they are often described as the dentine–pulp complex. This complex is usually isolated from the oral environment by a protective layer of enamel in the crown, and cementum in the root (Fig. 2.1). When these natural protective layers are lost, the dentine–pulp complex can be exposed to irritants and respond in different ways. The presence of dentinal tubules and their contents ensures that stimuli applied to dentine often also exert effects on the underlying pulp. Therefore, the complex responds to external stimuli as a continuum.

The pulp is anatomically divided into the coronal pulp (present in the pulp chamber), and the radicular pulp (located in the root canal). The radicular pulp communicates with the periodontal ligament directly via apical and lateral foramina (Fig. 2.1). As a consequence, pathological changes in the pulp tissue may affect the periapical tissues (periodontal ligament, alveolar bone and cementum). This chapter deals with the physiological, pathological, and microbiological aspects of the dentine–pulp complex and their effects on the periapical tissues. Understanding the basic aspects of the endodontic science is crucial for excellence in clinical practice.

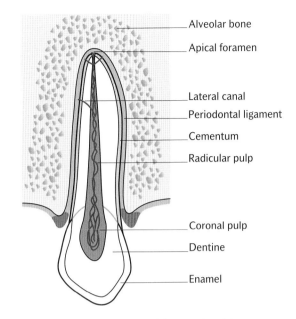

Figure 2.1 Structure of the tooth and the associated tissues.

Embryology of the dentine–pulp complex

The tooth derives from two basic embryonic cell types: the ectoderm, which forms the enamel, and the neural crest-derived ectomesenchyme, which forms the dentine, pulp, and periodontal tissues. The tooth starts to form during the 6th week of embryonic life as a localized thickening of the oral ectoderm associated with the embryonic maxillary and mandibular processes. This epithelial outgrowth leads to formation of the dental lamina. The subsequent process of tooth development is divided into three sequential stages, which are named according to the morphology of the developing tooth germ: (a) bud, (b) cap, and (c) bell. Initially, the tooth germ assumes the shape of a 'bud', as a result of proliferation of the epithelium from the dental lamina into the ectomesenchyme (Fig. 2.2a). Further continued epithelial proliferation gives origin to the enamel organ which forms a concavity that looks like a 'cap' (Fig. 2.2b). As the tooth germ enlarges and the invagination becomes deeper, the developing tooth assumes a shape resembling a 'bell'. The tissue located within the invagination is known as the dental papilla, which will ultimately give rise to the dentine and pulp. During the bell stage, the cells of the inner layer of the enamel organ differentiate into ameloblasts. Next, the cells in the outer layer of the dental papilla differentiate into odontoblasts, which start to produce the mantle dentine.

Root formation begins when cells of both inner and outer enamel epithelium converge to form the cervical loop, which demarcates the anatomic terminus of the crown and the point where the root starts to form. The fused epithelia give rise to the Hertwig´s epithelial sheath, which guides and initiates root formation by providing signals for the differentiation of odontoblasts and further dentine production. Following deposition of the first dentine layer in the root, the basement membrane beneath the Hertwig´s epithelial sheath disrupts. The cells of the innermost layer of the sheath then secrete a hyaline material over the newly formed dentine—the hyaline layer of Hopewell–Smith. This layer will be important to help the cementum to bind the radicular dentine.

After dentine is deposited, the Hertwig´s epithelial sheath fragments, and cells of the dental sac contact the formed dentine and differentiate into cementoblasts. Cementoblasts lay down acellular cementum over the hyaline layer. In sequence, bundles of collagen called Sharpey´s fibres are produced by fibroblasts in the central region of the dental sac and become embedded in the forming cementum. Concurrently, cells in the outermost area of the dental sac differentiate into osteoblasts and start to produce bone that will anchor the periodontal ligament fibres. Fibroblasts then produce more collagen that will form the principal periodontal ligament fibres. Undifferentiated mesenchymal stem cells abound in the periodontal ligament and hold the capacity to differentiate into the main matrix-producing cells of the periapical tissues, i.e. fibroblasts, cementoblasts, and osteoblasts.

Dentine

Composition

Dentine is a mineralized tissue that makes up the bulk of the tooth. By weight, it is composed of 70 per cent inorganic material (predominantly hydroxyapatite crystals), 20 per cent organic matrix, comprised mostly of collagen (about 90 per cent), and 10 per cent water. Collagen type I is the most abundant, but type V may also be found as a minor component. The dentine organic matrix also contains many growth

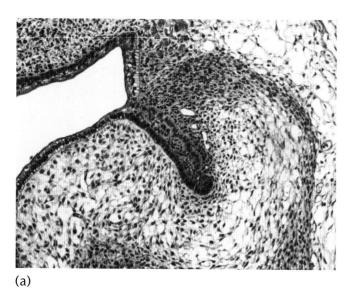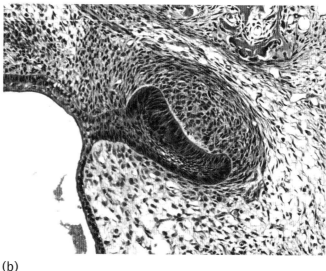

(a)   (b)

Figure 2.2 Initial stages of tooth development: (a) bud stage and (b) cap stage.

factors, including: transforming growth factor (TGF)-β, platelet-derived growth factor (PDGF), insulin-like growth factors (IGF) and bone morphogenetic proteins (BMPs). These growth factors are bound to the dentine matrix during dentinogenesis, but can be released during dentine dissolution processes (e.g. carious lesions), and thereby contribute to reparative events, including stimulation of tertiary dentine formation.

Types of dentine

There are different types of dentine (Fig. 2.3):

- *Mantle dentine* is the first dentine to be formed and is located immediately adjacent to enamel or cementum.
- *Primary dentine* is deposited during physiological dentine formation by odontoblasts and forms the bulk of the tooth.
- *Predentine* is a 10–40 μm wide zone of unmineralized dentine located between the odontoblast layer and the mineralized dentine.
- During dentinogenesis, odontoblasts move in a centripetal direction, leaving their cell processes within the dentine to form the *dentinal tubules* (Fig. 2.4). The odontoblast process extends up to one-third to one-half of the dentinal tubule.
- Dentine lining the tubules is known as *intratubular* (peritubular) dentine. The dentine located between the intratubular dentine constitutes the main bulk of dentine and is termed *intertubular* dentine. Intratubular dentine is more calcified and harder than the intertubular dentine.
- *Secondary dentine* is formed physiologically after the root is completely formed and the apex has reached its final stage of development. Secondary dentine is deposited by the existing odontoblasts at a lower rate than primary dentine.
- *Tertiary dentine* is formed in response to external stimuli (e.g., caries, microleakage). It is deposited beneath the site of injury, and the deposition rate is proportional to the degree of injury. Tertiary dentine can be categorized as reactionary and reparative dentine.

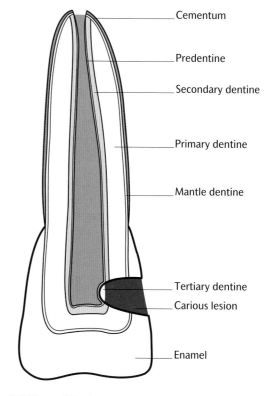

Figure 2.3 Types of dentine.

- *Reactionary dentine* is formed by odontoblasts that survived the injury and exhibit tubules that remain continuous with those from secondary dentine.
- *Reparative dentine* is formed by newly differentiated odontoblast-like cells, which originate from mesenchymal pulp stem cells. In reparative dentine, tubules (if present) are not continuous with those from secondary dentine.
- *Sclerotic dentine* comprises a partial or complete obliteration of the dentinal tubules and can result either from the increased production

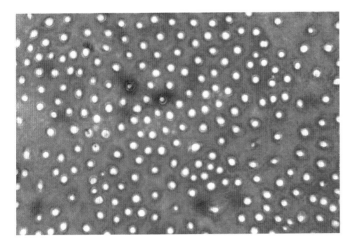

Figure 2.4 Dentinal tubules in cross-section.

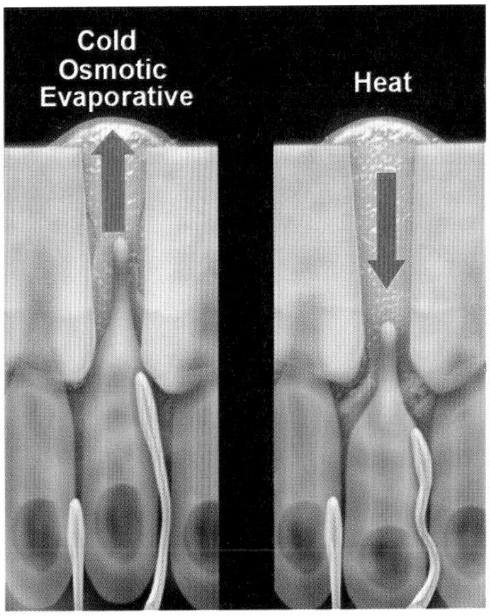

Figure 2.5 Hydrodynamic theory for dentine sensitivity. External stimuli cause inward or outward movement of the dentinal fluid and consequent mechanical distortion and activation of sensory nerve fibres.

of intratubular dentine or precipitation of hydroxyapatite and whit-lockite crystals within the tubules. Both tertiary and sclerotic dentine can be very important defensive mechanisms of the dentine–pulp complex to external injury.

Dentinal tubules

Dentinal tubules traverse the entire width of dentine with the largest diameter located near the pulp (about 2.5 μm), and the smallest diameter near the enamel or cementum (about 1 μm). The tubular density is also higher near the pulp, with about 65,000 tubules/mm² at the pulpal border, as compared to about 15,000 tubules/mm² at the enamel–dentine junction (EDJ). The area occupied by the dentinal tubules ranges from 1 per cent (at the EDJ) to 30 per cent (near the pulp). Tubules associated with a vital pulp contain the dentinal fluid, odontoblastic process, nerve endings (up to 100 μm deep), type I collagen, proteoglycans, and other proteins.

Permeability and sensitivity

The tubular structure provides dentine with two important properties: *permeability* and *sensitivity*. Because of dentine permeability, any substance applied to dentine has the potential to affect the pulp. Dentine permeability depends on several important physical factors including dentine diffusional surface area, dentine thickness, proximity to the

pulp, and the characteristics of the solute (size, charge, concentration, and water and lipid solubility). Since both the density and diameter of the tubules increase with depth, the permeability of dentine increases substantially near the pulp. The presence of smear layer (1–5 μm layer of dentinal debris formed after cutting dentine) and the degree of tubule occlusion (e.g. due to sclerosis) also influence permeability.

Dentine sensitivity is also related to the presence of tubules. Several theories have been suggested to explain the mechanisms of dentine sensitivity; the most accepted is the 'hydrodynamic theory'. This theory postulates that dentine responds to stimuli with pain due to the abrupt inward or outward movement of the dentinal tubule fluid induced by an external stimulus (Fig. 2.5). The rapid dentinal fluid displacement caused by pain-producing stimuli, such as: heat and cold (thermal stimuli), sweets (osmotic stimulus), probing and chewing (mechanical stimuli), and air blasts (evaporative stimulus), leads to displacement of odontoblasts. This gives rise to mechanical deformation and consequent activation of the sensory nerve terminals of low-threshold A-δ fibres located in close contact with odontoblasts.

Pulp

Functions

The main functions of the pulp are:

- **Formative**—the pulp is responsible for dentinogenesis;
- **Sensitivity**—pulp sensory innervation acts as an effective 'warning system'. For example, pain will not be experienced in a pulpless tooth until substantial damage has occurred in the tooth structure and the periapical tissues have been affected;

- **Nutrition**—pulp vascularization supplies oxygen and nutrients, which are essential for dentine formation and pulp survival itself;
- **Defence**—the pulp tissue can defend itself against microbial infection by producing sclerotic or tertiary dentine and mounting an immune response. Teeth with vital pulps are much more resistant to microbial infection and do not develop periapical periodontitis. Consequently, maintaining a vital pulp can be regarded as the best way to prevent periapical periodontitis.

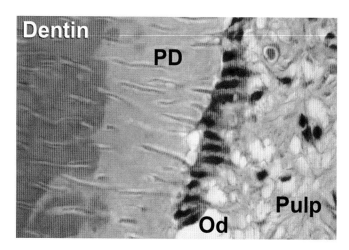

Figure 2.6 Odontoblasts (Od) forming a layer in the periphery of the pulp. These cells are the characteristic cells of the pulp. Predentine (PD).

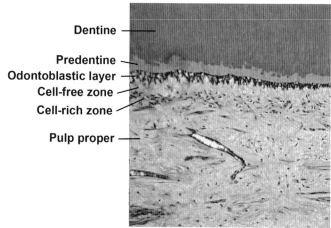

Figure 2.8 Morphologic zones of the pulp. The odontoblast layer is the most peripheral zone, lining the predentine. A high density of cells, including fibroblasts, undifferentiated stem cells and immune cells, forms the cell-rich zone region. The cell-free zone (zone of Weil) contains blood capillaries and a rich network of nerve fibres (Rashkow´s nervous plexus). The pulp proper is the central mass of the pulp tissue and contains the largest blood vessels and nerves, along with fibroblasts and other cells.

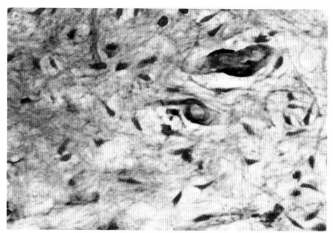

Figure 2.7 Fibroblasts in the pulp. These cells are the most abundant cells of the pulp tissue.

Composition

The pulp is a soft connective tissue composed of cells, extracellular connective matrix, blood vessels, and nerves. The odontoblast is the most characteristic cell of the dentine–pulp complex. Odontoblasts are organized as a single layer of cells (the odontoblast layer) at the borderline between dentine and pulp (Fig. 2.6). The cell body of the odontoblast is located in the pulp adjacent to the predentine. The cell also possesses a cytoplasmic projection (odontoblast process) left behind from dentinogenesis to form the dentinal tubule. Odontoblasts are postmitotic cells, and therefore cannot undergo further cell division. These cells are columnar in shape and more numerous in the coronal pulp; and flattened and less numerous in the radicular pulp. The other cells present in the pulp include: fibroblasts, undifferentiated mesenchymal stem cells, and various immune cells (macrophages, dendritic cells, lymphocytes). Fibroblasts are the most abundant cell type in the pulp (Fig. 2.7). Undifferentiated mesenchymal stem cells occur throughout

the pulp tissue, being more abundant in the pulp proper region. They have the ability to differentiate into odontoblast-like cells in response to injury and stimulation. The pulpal extracellular matrix is primarily produced by fibroblasts and consists of collagens and non-collagenous proteins. Collagen types I and III comprise the huge majority of the total collagen in the pulp tissue. The histological zones of the pulp tissue are shown in Fig. 2.8.

Vascularization

Pulp vascularization is provided by blood vessels that enter the pulp via apical foramen or foramina, and then extend and branch coronally. The pulp blood supply originates from branches of the infraorbital artery, the posterior superior alveolar artery, or the inferior alveolar artery, which in turn originate from the maxillary artery (Fig. 2.9). Once they enter the root canal, arterioles run longitudinally toward the coronal pulp, while capillaries branch off at right angles to form a dense capillary network at the periphery of the pulp (Fig. 2.10). Blood then drains into venules, which occupy a greater area in the central portion of the pulp. Pulp microcirculation also includes arteriovenous anastomoses, venous–venous anastomoses, and the U-turn loop arterioles, all of which may participate in the regulation of blood flow. Unlike most vascularized tissues in the body, the pulp lacks a true collateral blood supply, which makes this tissue more susceptible to the deleterious effects of severe inflammation. In addition, because the pulp is encased by the hard dentinal walls its volume cannot expand significantly under conditions of increased tissue pressure. This may influence pulp survival during an inflammatory event. The confines of the pulp chamber are known as a low-compliance environment.

The primary function of the microcirculation in any tissue is to supply oxygen and nutrients to resident cells, and remove waste products

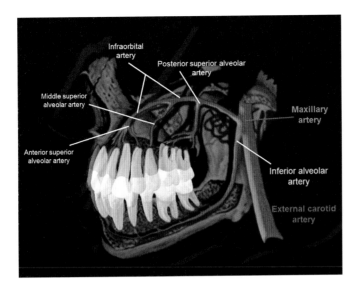

Figure 2.9 Vascular supply of the pulp and periapical tissues.

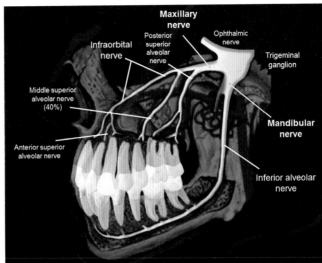

Figure 2.11 Sensory innervation of the pulp and periapical tissues originates from the maxillary and mandibular divisions of the trigeminal nerve.

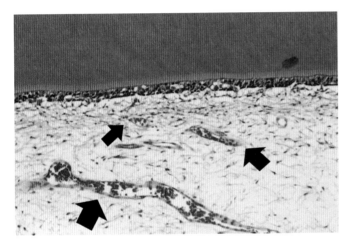

Figure 2.10 Blood vessels (arrows) in the peripheral pulp.

and carbon dioxide. The volume of pulp tissue occupied by blood vessels in the coronal pulp is about 14 per cent. Conceivably, the pulp has the highest blood flow value per unit weight of tissue among the oral tissues. Tissue pressure in the normal pulp has been estimated to be about 6–11 mmHg. This relatively high pulp tissue pressure leads to an outward flow of fluid in the dentinal tubules when dentine is exposed, helping to dilute bacterial products and counteract bacterial invasion of the vital pulp via tubules.

Innervation

The pulp has both sensory and autonomic innervation. Sensory innervation of the pulp and periapical tissues originates from the maxillary and mandibular divisions of the trigeminal nerve (Fig. 2.11). Trigeminal sensory neurons have a primary afferent projection that terminates as free nerve endings in the pulp and periodontal tissues. Approximately 1,000–2,000 nerves enter a single tooth—80 per cent of them are unmyelinated

(C fibres and sympathetic nerves) and 20 per cent are myelinated fibres (A fibres). Pulp nerves usually follow the blood vessels as they extend coronally and branch. At the subodontoblastic cell-free zone, nerve fibres give rise to a rich network of terminal endings to form the Rashkow´s nervous plexus.

The pulp tissue is innervated by three different trigeminal sensory nerve fibres: A-β fibres, A-δ fibres and C fibres (Table 2.1). A-β nerve fibres are myelinated with a very fast conduction speed. They compose a small percentage of the myelinated fibres (1–5%), and it is believed that they may be involved in nociception. A-δ nerve fibres are also myelinated, with rapid conduction speed and a low excitability threshold. A-δ fibres mediate the sharp, transient pain typical of dentine sensitivity. After leaving the Rashkow´s nervous plexus, A fibres lose their outer layer of Schwann cells and terminate as free nerve endings at the odontoblastic layer and the pulpal border of dentine. These fibres may enter some tubules and extend no more than 100 µm into coronal dentine and rarely do so in the radicular dentine. The sensory nerve fibres are especially numerous near the pulp horn tips and consequently this area can be the most sensitive area of dentine. Myelinated innervation of the pulp does not reach full maturation and organization until the tooth is fully formed, which helps explain why the pulps of young teeth are less responsive to sensitivity tests than those from adult teeth.

C fibres are unmyelinated, with a slow conduction speed and high excitability threshold. Stimulation of C fibres produces pain that is dull, aching, excruciating, often diffuse symptoms which is typical of irreversible pulpitis. Severe inflammation can cause increased tissue pressure and decrease in oxygen content, which may block conduction of nerve impulses in A-δ fibres, but not the C fibres.

Sympathetic nerve fibres can also be found in the pulp and originate from the superior cervical ganglion. They are involved with neurogenic modulation of the microcirculation and may have a role in dentinogenesis.

Table 2.1 Characteristics of different nerve fibre types found in dental pulp

Fibre	Function	Diameter (µm)	Conduction speed (m/sec)
Aβ	Pressure, touch	5–12	30–70
Aδ	Pain, temperature, touch	1–5	6–30
C	Pain	0.4–1	0.5–2
Sympathetic	Postganglionic sympathetic	0.3–1.3	0.7–2.3

Dentine–pulp response to caries

Caries is the most common cause of irritation to the dentine–pulp complex (Fig. 2.12). Once dentine is exposed as a result of destruction of enamel or cementum by caries, dentinal tubules may act as channels for bacterial products to diffuse toward the pulp border. As a biologic continuum, dentine and pulp respond to the bacterial stimuli from caries basically by three main mechanisms: (a) reduction in dentine permeability; (b) tertiary dentine formation; and (c) immune response (Fig. 2.13). The first two responses involve dentine and are intended to reinforce the barriers against bacterial invasion, providing additional protection to the pulp. All three responses usually develop concurrently and their intensity is directly proportional to the advancing caries process. Because caries can progress either rapidly or slowly, or can become inactive (arrested caries), the dentine–pulp complex response will vary accordingly.

Reduction in dentine permeability

Reduction in dentine permeability is an important defence mechanism against bacterial progress toward the pulp. In vital teeth, outward movement of dentinal fluid and the presence of vital tubular contents can conceivably delay intratubular invasion by bacteria. Moreover, the pulp can contribute to reduction of dentine permeability by increasing the outward fluid flow, lining tubules with proteins, and depositing sclerotic dentine. Host defence molecules, such as antibodies and components of the complement system, may be present in the dentinal fluid of vital teeth and assist in the protection against deep bacterial invasion of dentine. Dentine sclerosis is a very important factor contributing to reduced permeability, and commonly occurs under carious lesions.

Tertiary dentine formation

Tertiary dentine is another protective mechanism against bacterial invasion—essentially the pulp retreats in response to the advancing carious lesion. Tertiary dentine can be reactionary or reparative. Bacteria present in the caries biofilm produce acids that demineralize dentine resulting in the release of bioactive molecules within the dentine matrix. Many of these bioactive molecules are growth factors that have the ability to stimulate formation of tertiary dentine.

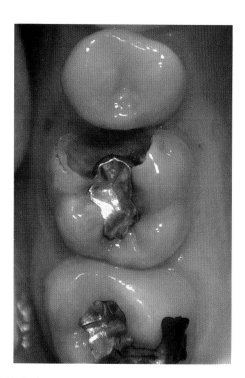

Figure 2.12 Carious lesion.

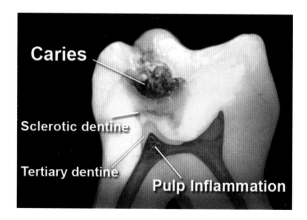

Figure 2.13 Basic mechanisms of dentine-pulp reaction to caries biofilm.

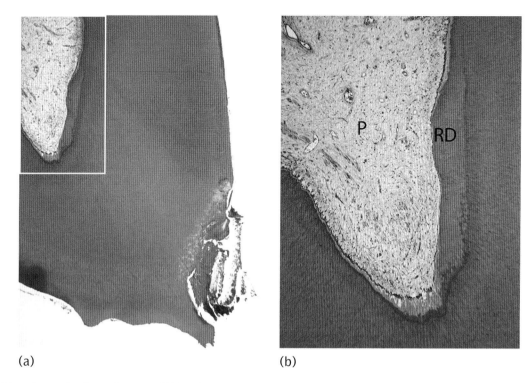

(a)   (b)

Figure 2.14 (a) Reactionary dentine under a superficial carious lesion and (b) higher magnification of outlined area ('P' pulp, 'RD' reactionary dentine').

Reactionary dentine is often formed under superficial or slowly progressing dentinal caries (Fig. 2.14a,b). Bacterial products released from the caries biofilm induce a focal upregulation of matrix production by odontoblasts, resulting in reactionary dentine formation. More advanced and aggressive carious lesions may lead to death of the subjacent odontoblasts. The tubules devoid of odontoblast cell processes are called dead tracts. Newly formed odontoblast-like cells deposit reparative dentine over the pulp side of the affected dentine, walling the highly permeable dead tracts off (Fig. 2.15). Therefore, whereas the reactionary dentine is produced by surviving original primary odontoblasts (Fig. 2.16), reparative dentine is produced by newly formed odontoblast-like cells originated from the undifferentiated mesenchymal stem cells (Fig. 2.17).

The amount of tertiary dentine formed in response to slowly progressing chronic caries is larger than that produced under rapidly advancing carious lesions. Reparative dentine commonly occurs in approximately two-thirds of teeth with caries, very often in association with dentine sclerosis.

Immune response—early inflammation

Like any other connective tissue in the body, the dental pulp responds to tissue injury by means of inflammation. Bacteria in caries biofilms represent the most common source of antigens and aggression toward the pulp. Pulpal inflammation develops as a low-grade response to caries (i.e. bacteria and their products) long before the pulp becomes directly exposed and infected. Bacterial products are diluted in the

dentinal fluid and travel the full tubule length to reach the pulp and elicit an inflammatory response.

Early pulpal inflammation in response to caries involves focal accumulation of chronic inflammatory cells underneath the affected dentine. Odontoblasts play an important role in this early response. Because they are the most peripherally located cells in the pulp, odontoblasts represent the first cells to encounter the carious bacterial products and the subsequent dentine matrix bioactive constituents released during demineralization. Odontoblasts can sense bacterial products and release proinflammatory molecules that recruit dendritic cells (and later other defence cells) to the pulp region subjacent to the affected dentine thus inducing an inflammatory response. As the caries progresses toward the pulp, the density of the chronic inflammatory infiltrate in the pulp increases.

Pulp innervation may participate in the defence response by a process referred to as neurogenic inflammation. By this process, afferent neurons respond to bacterial products by releasing neuropeptides, which are mediators that can attract host defence cells and induce vascular changes typical of inflammation.

The extent of pulp inflammation in response to caries depends on several factors, these include the depth of bacterial intratubular invasion, bacterial virulence, duration of the disease process and the degree to which dentine permeability was reduced. As for the depth of the carious lesion, it has been shown that when the distance between the advancing bacteria and the pulp is more than 1 mm, the intensity of the pulp inflammation is almost negligible. As the caries biofilm reaches

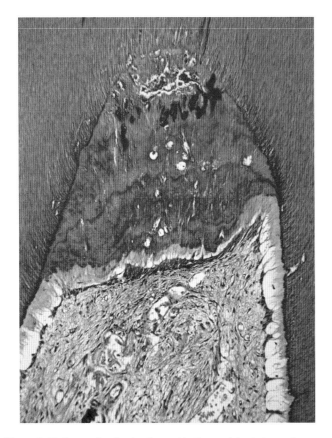

Figure 2.15 Reparative dentine formed in the mesial pulp horn of a mandibular first molar beneath a deep carious lesion. Note inclusions of necrotic tissue in the newly formed dentine.

to within 0.5 mm of the pulp, inflammation increases significantly, and becomes still more severe when the tertiary dentine formed beneath the caries is invaded by bacteria.

Even though the inflammatory response develops early in response to superficial caries, bacterial cells can be seen invading dentinal tubules to

some extent. However, the pulp tissue is not usually invaded by bacterial cells for as long as the pulp remains vital. Bacteria can reach the pulp via dentinal tubules even before a frank pulpal exposure, but they are not expected to cause irreversible damage to the pulp tissue. It is conceivable that vital pulp can eliminate these bacteria and clear or inactivate bacterial products.

Therefore, the pulp underneath a carious lesion rarely undergoes significant deleterious changes due to inflammation (e.g. abscess formation and necrosis), as long as the caries is confined to dentine. In these cases, pulp inflammation (pulpitis) is often regarded as reversible, because, in the event caries is removed or becomes inactive, pulp tissue repair can ensue. Caries removal and appropriate clinical management will generally lead to resolution of the inflammatory reaction, with reduction in the levels of defence cells and proinflammatory mediators, setting the stage for further tissue repair.

From irreversible pulpitis to periapical periodontitis

If caries remains untreated and active, the pulp response shifts from *reversible* to *irreversible* pulpitis, then to *partial necrosis* and eventually to *total pulp necrosis*. Concomitantly, the frontline of infection advances toward the apical portion of the root canal to eventually affect the periapical tissues via apical or lateral foramina. This chain of events may occur asymptomatically or symptoms may arise at any stage. The time elapsed between pulp exposure and infection of the apical root canal is unpredictable, but it is usually a slow process that very often occurs by tissue increments.

Pulpitis usually shifts from a reversible to an irreversible state when the pulp becomes exposed by the caries process (Fig. 2.18a,b). As caries destroys dentine and approaches the pulp, the inflammatory response becomes increased in magnitude. In response to advancing caries, polymorphonuclear neutrophils (PMNs) are progressively attracted and accumulate in the subjacent pulp area. The inflammatory

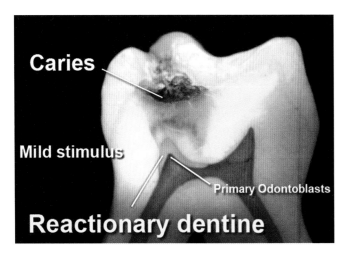

Figure 2.16 A superficial or slowly progressing dentinal carious lesion results in a relatively mild irritating stimulus that stimulates reactionary dentine formation by primary odontoblasts.

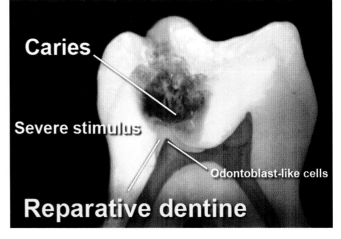

Figure 2.17 A deep or rapidly progressing dentinal carious lesion results in a severe irritating stimulus that causes death of primary odontoblasts and stimulates reparative dentine formation by odontoblast-like cells.

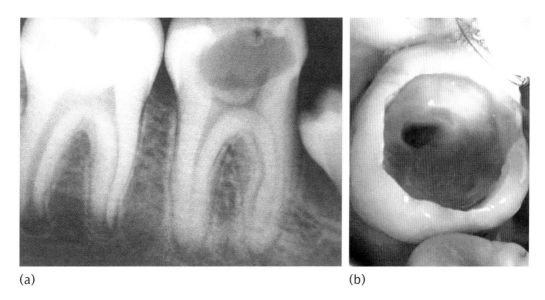

(a)   (b)

Figure 2.18 Carious pulp exposure: (a) radiographic findings and (b) clinical findings after caries excavation.

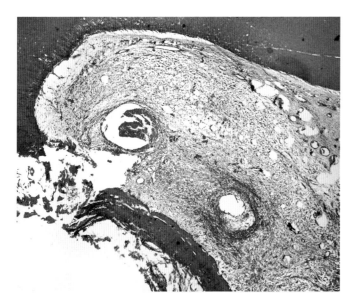

Figure 2.19 Histological section of a tooth with a carious exposure. The pulp was vital, but severely inflamed at the area of exposure.

Adapted from Siqueira J and Rôças I (2011) Case 1.1 Microbiology of primary periapical periodontitis. In: Patel S and Duncan H (eds) *Pitt Ford's Problem-Based Learning in Endodontology*, with permission from Wiley-Blackwell.

process becomes significantly exacerbated when the frontline of infection reaches the tertiary dentine. However, inflammation does not usually become severe to the point of being considered irreversible until the pulp is exposed.

When the pulp is eventually exposed, the tissue is in direct contact with a massive number of bacterial cells and their products from the caries biofilm. Direct exposure of the pulp to bacteria leads to severe acute inflammation in the tissue area subjected to bacterial aggression (Fig. 2.19). Typical vascular events take place, including vasodilation and increased vascular permeability, resulting in exudation. This leads to oedema formation, with consequent increase in tissue hydrostatic pressure, which can be critical for the pulp. Tissue pressure may eventually exceed that of thin-walled venules, which become compressed and collapse. Consequently, drainage is impeded and stagnation of blood flow not only promotes increased blood viscosity, but also impairs removal of waste products. This may lead to cell death and tissue necrosis.

As a consequence of intense acute vascular effects, PMNs continue to accumulate near the pulp exposure area. PMNs contribute to tissue damage by releasing enzymes and oxygen-derived radicals that degrade pulp tissue components. Bacterial products, such as enzymes, metabolites, and leukotoxins, also contribute to direct tissue damage. Localized abscesses may develop in the pulp adjacent to the exposed area.

This sequence of events occurs in the tissue area adjacent to the frontline of bacterial infection, but not in the entire extent of the pulp. Tissue pressure near the site of inflammation is almost normal and shows no signs of severe inflammation. This indicates that tissue pressure changes do not spread rapidly. A pressure difference of 8–10 mmHg has been measured between the inflamed and the non-inflamed adjacent area of the pulp, therefore significant pressure differences may be observed at sites only 1–2 mm apart. In the non-inflamed tissue area a few millimetres away from the inflamed area, tissue pressure is usually within normal range. This difference in pressure can be a result of several oedema-preventing mechanisms, which include lymphatics and the resilience of the ground substance of the pulp tissue.

Total pulp necrosis is a result of the gradual accumulation of local necrosis. After necrosis of pulp tissue, the frontline of bacterial infection gradually moves in an apical direction. Consequently, the tissue immediately adjacent to the infected region is injured and responds with the same inflammatory vascular events described above. Therefore, after pulp exposure to caries, pulp tissue compartments are subjected to a series of events: injury, inflammation, necrosis, and infection, which occur by tissue increments until the entire pulp is necrotic and infected. The inflammatory response to advancing endodontic infection can extend to the periodontal ligament even before the frontline of infection (and necrosis) reaches the apical or lateral foramina.

Periapical periodontitis is an inflammatory condition affecting the periapical tissues and can be usually regarded as a sequel to caries. This is because untreated caries can ultimately lead to pulp inflammation, necrosis, and infection. Development of periapical periodontitis is related to innate and adaptive immune responses to intraradicular bacterial infection in an attempt to contain the spread of the infection to the bone and other body sites.

The intensity of bacterial aggression toward the periapical tissues depends on the number of pathogenic bacteria and their virulence. These factors, counteracted by the host defences, can give rise to an acute inflammatory response (acute periapical periodontitis or acute apical abscess), or a chronic response (chronic periapical periodontitis). Chronic disease is usually characterized by bone destruction around the apex of the root (Fig. 2.20).

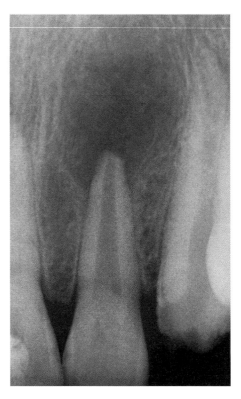

Figure 2.20 Periapical periodontitis associated with a maxillary incisor with a history of trauma. The periapical radiolucency represents bone destruction in response to intraradicular infection.

Endodontic infections

Routes of pulp invasion

Under normal conditions, the dentine–pulp complex is sterile and isolated from the oral microbiota by overlying enamel and cementum. In the event that the integrity of these natural layers is breached or naturally absent (Fig. 2.21), the dentine–pulp complex is exposed to the oral environment and then challenged by microbes present in carious lesions, in saliva bathing the exposed area, or in plaque biofilm that has formed on the exposed area. Microbes from sub-gingival biofilms associated with periodontal disease may also have access to the pulp via dentinal tubules at the cervical region of the tooth, and lateral/apical foramina. Microbes may also have access to the root canal at any time during or after professional endodontic intervention.

It is important to remember that whatever the route of microbial access to the root canal, necrosis of pulp tissue is a prerequisite for the establishment of primary endodontic infections. As discussed above, the vital pulp is highly competent in protecting itself against microbial invasion and colonization. However, if the pulp becomes necrotic as a result of caries, trauma, operative procedures, or periodontal disease, it can be easily infected because host defences no longer function therein.

Another situation in which the root canal system is devoid of host defences relates to teeth whose pulps were removed for treatment. Thus, microbes may also be introduced into the root canal space after endodontic treatment and cause a secondary infection. This may occur during endodontic treatment (due to a breach in asepsis, i.e. not using rubber dam), between appointments, or even after root canal filling (because of coronal leakage).

Types of endodontic infections

Endodontic infections are usually bacterial infections. Although other microbes, such as fungi, archaea, and virus have already been found in root canals of teeth associated with periapical periodontitis, bacteria are the most common microbes involved with this disease.

Endodontic infections can be classified according to the anatomical location as intraradicular or extraradicular infection. Intraradicular infection is caused by microbes colonizing the root canal system and can be subdivided into three categories according to the time microbes invaded the root canal system: primary, persistent, and secondary. Extraradicular infection develops as a sequel to intraradicular infection and is characterised by microbial invasion of the periapical tissues.

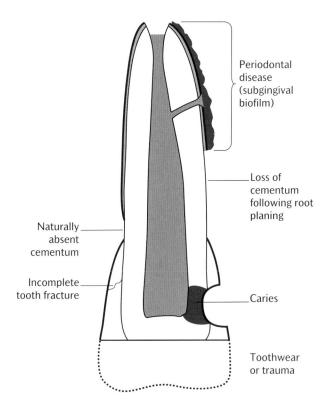

Periodontal disease (subgingival biofilm)

Loss of cementum following root planing

Naturally absent cementum

Incomplete tooth fracture

Caries

Toothwear or trauma

Figure 2.21 Routes of pulpal invasion.

Primary intraradicular infection

Primary intraradicular infection is caused by bacteria that initially invade and colonize the necrotic pulp tissue. Participating bacteria may have been involved in the earlier stages of pulp infection (usually from caries biofilms) or they can be latecomers that took advantage of the environmental conditions in the root canal after pulp necrosis.

Primary infections are characterized by a mixed community dominated by anaerobic bacteria. An infected root canal can harbour a mean of 10 to 20 bacterial species, which collectively reach a population density of about 10^3 to 10^8 bacterial cells. The size of this population is similar to some countries! Root canals of teeth associated with sinus tracts and/or large periapical radiolucencies usually harbour a heavy bacterial infection. Root canals of teeth with large periapical lesions may contain over 40 bacterial species.

Primary infections can be associated with either chronic or acute periapical periodontitis. Regardless of the presence of symptoms, the species frequently detected in primary infections belong to diverse genera of gram-negative and gram-positive bacteria (Table 2.2).

Culture methods have been traditionally used for identification of endodontic bacteria, but introduction of molecular microbiology methods that identify bacteria by their DNA or RNA has improved our knowledge of the bacterial diversity in endodontic infections. Molecular methods have also revealed that approximately 40–55 per cent of the bacteria found in root canals of teeth with periapical periodontitis still remain to be cultivated, named, and phenotypically characterized.

Acute periapical periodontitis and acute apical abscesses are the typical symptomatic forms of periapical periodontitis. In these cases, the infection is located in the root canal but it may also reach the periapical tissues and, specifically in abscessed cases, it has the potential to spread to other anatomical spaces of head and neck to form a cellulitis. Acute apical abscesses usually comprise a continuum of infection involving the root canal (intraradicular infection) and the periapical tissues (extraradicular infection).

The microbiota involved with abscesses is mixed and dominated by anaerobic bacteria. Bacterial counts per abscess case range from 10^4 to 10^9 colony-forming units. The mean number of species is comparatively higher in abscesses than in canals of teeth with chronic periapical periodontitis. Thus far, there is no strong evidence reporting on the specific involvement of a single species with any particular sign or symptom of periapical periodontitis.

Secondary and persistent intraradicular infections

Secondary intraradicular infection is caused by microbes that were not present in the primary infection, but were introduced in the root canal at any time after endodontic treatment was carried out (so-called because it is secondary to intervention). Secondary infections represent a contamination issue that may arise during (e.g. due to a breach in asepsis) or between appointments (e.g. due to coronal leakage), or even after endodontic treatment has been completed (e.g. due to coronal leakage).

Persistent intraradicular infection is caused by microbes that originated from the primary or secondary infection and that in some way resisted intracanal antimicrobial procedures and managed to endure periods of nutrient deprivation in treated canals. Persistent and secondary infections may cause clinical problems, including persistent exudation, persistent symptoms, inter-appointment exacerbations (flare-ups), and, ultimately, failure of the endodontic treatment.

In the clinical setting, it is virtually impossible to distinguish a persistent infection from a secondary infection. Exceptions include infectious complications (such as an apical abscess) arising after the treatment of non-infected vital pulps or cases in which periapical periodontitis was absent at the time of treatment but present in the follow-up radiograph, both of which represent typical examples of secondary infections.

Microbial species involved in secondary infections can be oral or non-oral microbes, depending on the source of contamination. If contamination comes from saliva leakage in the root canal, the microbes involved are normal oral inhabitants. On the other hand, the source of contamination can be non-oral, either from the environment (e.g. nosocomial infections) or from other body areas. Intracanal occurrence of *Pseudomonas aeruginosa*, *Staphylococcus species*, *Escherichia coli*, other enteric rods, *Candida* species, and *Enterococcus faecalis*, all of which are not usually found in primary infections, is highly suggestive of a secondary infection. Secondary infections can become persistent and cause post-treatment disease.

Teeth with post-treatment periapical periodontitis represent typical examples of persistent/secondary infections. The microbiota in endodontically treated teeth with periapical periodontitis exhibits a decreased diversity in comparison to primary infections. Well treated root canals typically harbour 1–5 species, while the number of species in inadequately treated root canals may reach up to 10–30 species, which is similar to untreated root canals. Bacterial counts in treated root canals vary from 10^3 to 10^7 cells.

Enterococcus faecalis, a facultative gram-positive coccus, has been the most frequently detected bacterial species in endodontically

Table 2.2 Bacterial genera and respective representative species commonly found in endodontic infections

Genus	Common cultivable species	Genus	Common cultivable species
Gram-negative		**Gram-positive**	
Anaerobic rods		Anaerobic rods	
Campylobacter	*C. rectus, C. gracilis*	*Actinomyces*	*A. israelii, A. odontolyticus*
Dialister	*D. invisus, D. pneumosintes*	*Eubacterium*	*E. infirmum, E. nodatum*
Fusobacterium	*F. nucleatum*	*Filifactor*	*F. alocis*
Porphyromonas	*P. endodontalis, P. gingivalis*	*Lactobacillus*	*L. catenaformis*
Prevotella	*P. intermedia, P. nigrescens, P. baroniae*	*Olsenella*	*O. uli*
Pyramidobacter	*P. piscolens*	*Propionibacterium*	*P. acnes, P. propionicum*
Tannerella	*T. forsythia*	*Pseudoramibacter*	*P. alactolyticus*
Anaerobic cocci		*Solobacterium*	*S. moorei*
Veillonella	*V. parvula*	Anaerobic cocci	
Anaerobicspirochaetes		*Parvimonas*	*P. micra*
Treponema	*T. denticola, T. socranskii, T. maltophilum*	*Peptostreptococcus*	*P. anaerobius*
		Streptococcus	*S. anginosus, S. constellatus, S. intermedius*
Facultative rods		Facultative rods	
Eikenella	*E. corrodens*	*Actinomyces*	*A. naeslundii*
Facultative cocci		Facultative cocci	
Neisseria	*N. mucosa*	*Enterococcus*	*E. faecalis*
		Streptococcus	*S. mitis, S. sanguinis, S. oralis*

treated teeth, with prevalence values reaching up to 90 per cent of the cases. This species is found in significantly lower prevalence in primary infections. *E. faecalis* has been commonly recovered from cases treated in multiple visits and/or in teeth left open for drainage, which suggests that it may be involved with a secondary infection. This species has been considered as transient in the oral cavity and its main source might be food or water.

Other bacteria found in endodontically treated teeth with periapical periodontitis include streptococci and some fastidious anaerobic bacterial species. As with primary infections, uncultivated bacteria are also found in treated root canals with post-treatment disease and may correspond to 55 per cent of the species detected.

Fungi are only occasionally found in primary infections, *Candida* species have been detected in endodontically treated teeth in up to 18 per cent of the retreatment cases. *Candida albicans* is by far the most commonly detected fungal species in endodontically treated teeth.

Extraradicular infection

Periapical periodontitis develops in response to intraradicular infection and for the most part comprises an effective barrier against spread of the infection to the alveolar bone and other body sites. In most situations, this inflammatory barrier manages to prevent bacteria from invading and establishing an infectious process in the periapical tissues. However, in some specific circumstances, bacteria

can overcome this defence barrier and give rise to an extraradicular infectious process. Extraradicular infection is characterized by microbial invasion of the inflamed periapical tissues and is a sequel to intraradicular infection.

The most common form of extraradicular infection is the acute apical abscess. There are, however, other forms of extraradicular infection that can be characterized by absence of acute symptoms. These conditions encompass the establishment of bacteria in the periapical tissues, either adhered to the apical external root surface in the form of extraradicular biofilms or forming cohesive actinomycotic colonies within the body of the inflammatory lesion (a condition known as apical actinomycosis). These types of extraradicular infections have been proposed as possible causes of post-treatment periapical periodontitis.

The prevalence of extraradicular infections in untreated teeth is low. Even in endodontically treated teeth with post-treatment disease, for which a higher frequency of extraradicular bacteria has been reported, a high rate of healing following retreatment is indirect evidence that the major cause of post-treatment disease is located within the root canal system, characterizing a persistent/secondary intraradicular infection. It is fair to assume that most cases of extraradicular infection are nurtured by a concomitant intraradicular infection. If the latter is properly controlled by root canal treatment, the former is expected to be effectively controlled by the host defences.

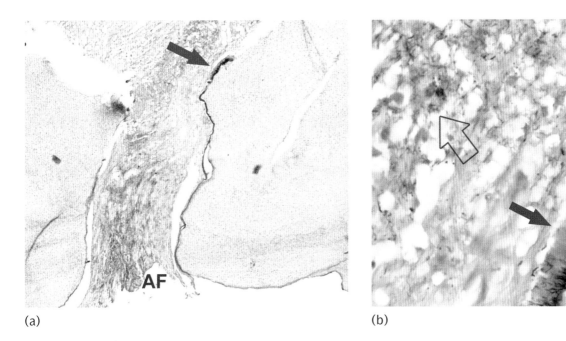

(a) (b)

Figure 2.22 Bacterial colonization of a necrotic root canal: (a) histological section of the apical portion of the root canal of a tooth affected by periapical periodontitis. A bacterial biofilm (arrow) is seen adhered to the root canal wall in close proximity to the apical foramen (AF) and (b) higher magnification of the biofilm. Planktonic bacterial cells are also seen in the main canal (empty arrow).

Adapted from Siqueira J and Rôças I (2011) Case 1.1 Microbiology of primary periapical periodontitis. In: Patel S and Duncan H (eds), *Pitt Ford's Problem-Based Learning in Endodontology*, with permission from Wiley-Blackwell.

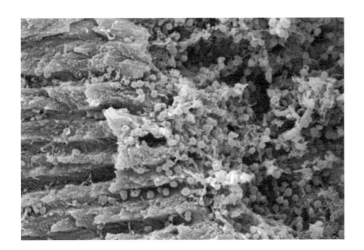

Figure 2.23 Bacterial cells colonizing the root canal wall and invading the dentinal tubules.

Virus infection and periapical periodontitis

Several herpesviruses and papillomavirus have been detected in periapical periodontitis lesions, where living host cells are present. It has been hypothesized that some herpesviruses, specifically human cytomegalovirus (HCMV) and Epstein–Barr virus (EBV), may be implicated in the pathogenesis of periapical periodontitis. It remains to be clarified whether these viruses participate in the pathogenesis of the periapical periodontitis, or their occurrence is just a epiphenomenon of bacterial infection and periapical inflammation.

Biofilms in endodontics

Like caries and marginal periodontitis, periapical periodontitis is a biofilm-induced disease. Most bacteria colonizing the root canal system usually grow as sessile biofilm communities that adhere to the dentinal walls, but flocks (bacterial aggregates/coaggregates) and planktonic cells also occur suspended in the fluid phase of the main root canal (Fig. 2.22). Lateral canals and isthmi connecting main canals can be clogged with bacteria, primarily organized in biofilms. Dentinal tubules underneath biofilm structures are often invaded by bacteria in about 70–80 per cent of root canals of teeth with periapical periodontitis (Fig. 2.23). A shallow intratubular penetration is more common, but bacterial cells may reach up to 300 μm deep in some teeth.

Bacterial biofilms are very prevalent in the apical portion of root canals of teeth with either primary or post-treatment periapical periodontitis. Endodontic biofilms present bacterial cells encased in an extracellular amorphous matrix and are often challenged by host inflammatory cells. Whereas intraradicular biofilms are common in teeth with periapical periodontitis, extraradicular biofilms are found much less frequently and usually in association with symptoms. Intraradicular bacterial biofilms are expected to be still more prevalent in the root canals of teeth associated with long-standing pathologic processes, including large apical radiolucencies and cysts. The very high frequency of biofilms in the root canals of endodontically treated teeth with post-treatment disease may be seen as indirect evidence that, depending on location and possibly species composition, biofilms can be a challenge for proper root canal disinfection.

Summary points

- Teeth undergo physiological and pathological changes through-out their life.

- There are several types of dentine. Primary dentine is deposited during physiological dentine formation. Secondary dentine is formed physiologically after the root is completely formed. Tertiary dentine is formed in response to external stimuli and may be *reactionary* or *reparative*.

- The pulp is a soft connective tissue composed of cells, extracellular connective matrix, blood vessels and nerves.

- The main functions of the pulp are formative, sensitivity, nutrition, and defence.

- Under normal circumstances the dentine–pulp complex is sterile. In the event that the protective enamel and cemental coverings are lost or absent, the dentine–pulp complex can become challenged by microbes from the oral cavity.

- Pathological changes in dentine may affect the pulp and in turn may affect the periapical tissues. Responses include pulpal inflammation, pulpal necrosis, and periapical periodontitis.

- Endodontic infections are primarily bacterial in nature. These bacteria grow as a biofilm community that adheres to dentinal walls. Endodontic infections may be intraradicular (primary, secondary or persistent) or extraradicular infections.

 Suggested further reading

Baumgartner JC (2004) Microbiologic aspects of endodontic infections. *Journal of California Dental Association* **32**, 459–68.

Cooper PR, Takahashi Y, Graham LW, Simon S, Imazato S and Smith AJ (2010) Inflammation-regeneration interplay in the dentine–pulp complex. *Journal of Dentistry* **38**, 687–97.

Figdor D and Gulabivala K (2008) Survival against the odds: microbiology of root canals associated with post-treatment disease. *Endodontic Topics* **18**, 62–77.

Holland GR and Torabinejad M (2009) The dental pulp and periradicular tissues. In: Torabinejad M and Walton RE (eds) *Endodontics: Principles and practice*, 4th edn; pp. 1–20. St. Louis, MO, USA: Saunders Elsevier.

Nanci A (2008) *Ten Cate's Oral Histology: development, structure, and function*, 7th edn. St. Louis, MO, USA: Mosby Elsevier.

Pashley DH (1996) Dynamics of the pulpo–dentin complex. *Critical review in oral biology and medicine* **7**, 104–33.

Ricucci D and Siqueira JF Jr (2010) Biofilms and apical periodontitis: study of prevalence and association with clinical and histopathologic findings. *Journal of Endodontics* **36**, 1277–88.

Siqueira JF Jr and Rôças IN (2008) Clinical implications and microbiology of bacterial persistence after treatment procedures. *Journal of Endodontics* **34**, 1291–1301.

Siqueira JF Jr and Rôças IN (2009) Community as the unit of pathogenicity: an emerging concept as to the microbial pathogenesis of apical periodontitis. *Oral Surgery, Oral Medicine, Oral Pathology, Oral Radiology, and Endodontics* **107**, 870–8.

Siqueira JF Jr and Rôças IN (2009) Diversity of endodontic microbiota revisited. *Journal of Dental Research* **88**, 969–81.

Sundqvist G and Figdor D (2003) Life as an endodontic pathogen. Ecological differences between the untreated and root-filled root canals. *Endodontic Topics* **6**, 3–28.

Online Resource Centre

 To help you to develop and apply your knowledge and skills further, we have provided interactive learning resources online at http://www.oxfordtextbooks.co.uk/orc/patel/

3

Diagnosis, treatment planning, and patient management

Bun San Chong,
Justin J. Barnes,
Shanon Patel

Chapter contents

What is diagnosis?

This section will introduce the rationale for diagnosis. It is important that you read the whole chapter to understand how the theory and practice of diagnosis are related.

Diagnosis is the process in which a disease, abnormality, or complaint is identified by collecting and analysing information on the presenting symptoms, clinical signs, and the results of specific investigations or tests. *An accurate diagnosis is the key to successful treatment.* The importance of the process cannot be over-emphasized. A correct diagnosis serves not only to confirm but also exclude other causative factors. The treatment options available and the planned management of the patient are dependent on a correct diagnosis.

It is not uncommon for a patient to have self-diagnosed their problem as being of dental origin and expects immediate and effective treatment. However, the clinician should always maintain an open mind when considering a patient's complaint. The possibility of other (including non-dental) causes, should always be borne in mind. The question: 'Is this a dental problem or not?' should always be asked when making a diagnosis.

In general, endodontic diagnosis involves identifying the state of pulpal and periapical health, in order to arrive at a suitable treatment plan. It should always take into account the patient as an individual, the potential technical difficulties associated with treatment that may be encountered, and the clinician's competence. Some of the initial questions that should be asked include:

- Is the complaint related to a dental cause?
- Are the symptoms pulpal and/or periodontal in origin?
- Is the presentation suggestive of a healthy pulp or not?
- Is it possible to manage and treat this patient successfully?

If a complaint of pain does not appear to be associated with teeth, i.e. non-odontogenic, it is necessary to consider other causes of orofacial pain (Table 3.1). If a definitive diagnosis cannot be established, or if the patient's complaint is not dental in origin, referral to an appropriate specialist may be indicated. In addition, until and unless there is a definitive diagnosis, it is prudent to be cautious and irreversible treatment should not be carried out.

A sound diagnosis can only be reached when information is collected from the patient in a systematic and meticulous manner (Table 3.2). The information can then be interpreted and acted upon accordingly. Each step of the diagnostic process is aimed at:

- Gaining the relevant and the maximum information regarding the complaint;

Table 3.1 Examples of non-dental causes of orofacial pain

Source	Examples
Extraoral	Salivary glands, sinuses, lymphatic system
Musculoskeletal	Temporomandibular disorders, masticatory muscle disorders
Neuropathic	Trigeminal neuralgia, atypical odontalgia, post-herpetic neuralgia
Neurovascular	Tension-type headaches, migraine, cluster headaches
Psychogenic	Major depressive disorders, anxiety disorders

Table 3.2 The stages involved in reaching a diagnosis

Patient history
- Presenting complaint
- History of the presenting complaint
- Dental history
- Medical history
- Personal history

Examination of the patient
- Extraoral
- Intraoral

Special investigations
- Sensibility testing
- Radiographic examination

- Providing help and guidance towards additional tests or further investigations;
- Corroborating the evidence as to the likely cause(s) of the complaint.

When the information from one aspect of the diagnostic procedure does not tally with the results from another aspect of the diagnostic procedure(s), it may mean that further investigations are required and/or the information collected so far may be incorrect and/or insufficient. Diagnostic errors usually arise when the process is not performed in a systematic and methodical manner or some of the steps have been missed. For example, if the clinical examination is only cursory, this may lead to the clinician choosing the wrong investigations and, more crucially, the formulation of an incorrect treatment plan.

What are the aims of history taking?

The primary aim of history taking is to gain as much relevant information as possible from the patient to arrive at an initial provisional diagnosis. It is, therefore, important to ask appropriate questions and listen carefully to what the patient has to say. History taking also aims to:

- Guide the clinician in deciding what to concentrate on during examination and what special investigations will be necessary to confirm a diagnosis.
- Establish a rapport with the patient.

- Gain insight into the patient's motivations and assess the patient's expectations from dental treatment.
- Reveal any potential complications that may dictate the need to modify the treatment plan.

The amount of useful information gleaned from the patient will vary and is dependent on several factors. These include the patient's ability to convey or describe the symptoms experienced and its accuracy; the severity of the distress, discomfort or pain, and the impact of the symptoms on the patient. At times, a patient may present with more than one complaint. In these situations, it is prudent to concentrate on each complaint separately according to their seriousness or urgency.

This section will focus on aspects of history taking that are of direct relevance to endodontics.

Presenting complaint

The diagnostic process starts with asking the patient why they are seeking dental care. The opening question should be simple and to the point, for example: 'How can I help you?'. The patient's presenting complaint should be in their own words. Endodontic presenting complaints commonly include pain/discomfort, swelling, discharge, bad taste, and/or tooth discolouration. The history of the presenting complaint should then be explored to find out how long the patient has been suffering, and if or how the symptoms have changed with time.

Dental history

The aim of the dental history is to gain an insight into what previous dental treatment has been carried out, as well as the patient's attitudes towards dental treatment and their own teeth.

Attendance

It is useful to know about the past dental history to establish whether the patient is a regular attender or only attends when in pain. A patient in the latter category may be less motivated. If pain is the reason for seeking a second opinion, it is worthwhile establishing whether the presenting complaint may be related to recent dental treatment with another dentist. The patient should be asked for details about any dental treatment recently received.

Oral hygiene and dietary habits

The patient's oral hygiene and dietary habits should be noted. The level of sugar consumption and the acidic components in their diet should also be determined. Key questions may help in elucidating causal factors related to the patient's complaint. For example, a patient with a 'sweet tooth' will be more susceptible to caries, which may, eventually, lead to pulpal involvement.

Previous trauma

It may be pertinent to ask the patient if there is a past history of dental trauma related to the tooth in question. Dental trauma more frequently involves anterior rather than posterior teeth. For example, pulpal necrosis or discolouration of an unrestored anterior tooth may have been caused by previous traumatic injury such as a sports-related accident (Fig. 3.1).

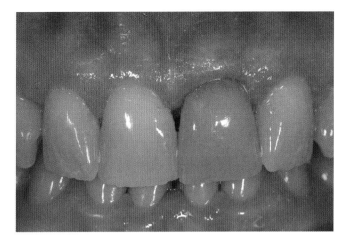

Figure 3.1 Discoloured maxillary central incisor with a history of trauma.

Medical history

The aim of the medical history is to ascertain if there are any medical conditions that may directly or indirectly influence patient management. It is, therefore, essential that the medical history is thorough and up-to-date. If there are any uncertainties or queries about the general health of the patient, or if it is likely to have an impact on treatment, it is advisable to liaise with the patient's general medical practitioner or their medical consultant.

Although there are no medical conditions which strictly contraindicate endodontic treatment, there are some conditions that may modify the endodontic management. Common medical problems that may influence or require modification of the treatment plan include:

- Blood dyscrasias or anticoagulation therapy;
- Recent history of myocardial infarction;
- Immunocompromised patients;
- Steroid treatment or recent history of steroid treatment;
- Bisphosphonate treatment or history of bisphosphonate treatment;
- High-risk patients, e.g. Hepatitis C, HIV;
- Poorly controlled diabetes;
- History of depression or psychiatric illness;
- Pregnancy;
- Allergies.

Often, the patient's medical history may only be an issue depending on the type of treatment required. For example, non-surgical endodontic treatment of a patient on anticoagulant therapy rarely presents problems. However, if the patient requires surgical endodontics then the anticoagulant therapy may have to be altered. A patient who is on or has been on bisphosphonates is another example; in these cases, extraction, even of a very compromised tooth, may be inadvisable and endodontic treatment may be the treatment of choice.

Before prescribing any type of medication as part of dental treatment, it is essential that checks are made on possible interactions with any medication the patient may be taking. A note should also be made of any antibiotics (including dosage, frequency, and duration) the patient may have taken recently, as this may influence the prescription of further antibiotics that may become necessary. Specific questions regarding allergy to latex, household bleach, and iodine compounds, for example, should be asked as these materials and chemicals are commonly used in endodontic treatment.

Previously, patients considered at risk of infective endocarditis undergoing interventional procedures were given antibiotic prophylaxis. As a result, patients with a wide range of cardiac conditions including a history of rheumatic fever, were prescribed this preventative measure. However, the current medical consensus is that there is little evidence to support this empirical practice. Antibiotic prophylaxis has not been proven to be effective and there is no clear association between episodes of infective endocarditis and interventional procedures. In addition, any benefits from prophylaxis need to be weighed against the risks of adverse effects for the patient and of antibiotic resistance developing.

Following newer guidelines issued by the National Institute for Health and Clinical Excellence (NICE), antibiotic prophylaxis should no longer be routinely offered for defined interventional procedures. It is advisable to liaise with the patient's general medical practitioner or their cardiac specialist if clarification on the need for antibiotic prophylaxis is required.

Personal history

It is useful to obtain an insight into the patient's personal and professional lifestyles as there may be clues to possible contributory or aetiological factors that may have a bearing on the presenting complaint. A classic example is pain from temporomandibular dysfunction, initiated or aggravated by episodes of stress in a patient's personal or professional life, which may be mistaken for an endodontic problem. Patients should also be asked if they think or know that they clench their teeth during the day and/or while they sleep.

What are the aims of the extraoral examination?

In the dental context, the aims of the extraoral examination are to assess the head and neck region whilst looking for signs that may be related to pulpal or periapical diseases; for example, a facial swelling. The muscles of mastication, lymph glands, and temporomandibular joints may also be assessed.

What are the aims of the intraoral examination?

The aims of the intraoral examination are to gain a general view of the mouth, and then a specific view of the area(s) of the main complaint. The intraoral examination should be sufficiently detailed to detect signs of non-endodontic and endodontic disease. It is also important to assess the patient's tolerance of dentistry.

What are the aims of special investigations?

Special investigations or tests are needed to corroborate or exclude initial findings and to obtain further information of relevance. They may also be used to identify or confirm the provisional diagnosis by helping to reproduce the reported symptoms. The commonest special investigations carried out are sensibility testing and radiographic examination.

Sensibility testing

The aim of sensibility testing (traditionally referred to as vitality testing), is to attempt to assess the health of the pulp. As it is reliant on the responsiveness of the nerve supply to the applied stimulus (electric or thermal), sensibility testing equipment can only provide an indication but not an absolute confirmation of pulpal health. Sensibility testing assumes that the status of the nerve supply of the tooth is a reflection of the status of the blood supply. It is important to be aware that sensibility testing may provide false positive, as well as false negative results.

A positive response is usually due to stimulation of Aδ nerve fibres by the electric stimulus or contraction/expansion of the fluid within the dentinal tubules by thermal stimulus. If the sensation disappears quickly (within 10–15 seconds) following removal of the stimulus, this is considered to indicate that the pulp–dentine complex is healthy. When a lingering dull ache persists following the removal of the stimulus, suggesting that there has been stimulation of the C fibres, this is considered indicative of irreversible pulpal inflammation. No response from pulp testing indicates that the tooth is non-vital, i.e. the pulp is necrotic.

Radiographic examination

Preoperative periapical radiographs should always be taken as part of the diagnostic process. Periapical radiographs are usually the most valuable radiographic views of the teeth and their surrounding periapical structures.

Periapical radiographs may reveal clues about the status of the pulp. There may be obvious signs of pulpal involvement; for example, a periapical radiolucency (Fig. 3.2) or evidence of gross caries (Fig. 3.3). However, more subtle signs of pulpal involvement include the presence of tertiary dentine, calcified root canals, widening of the periodontal ligament space and root resorption. Periapical radiographs may also reveal signs indicative of a vertical

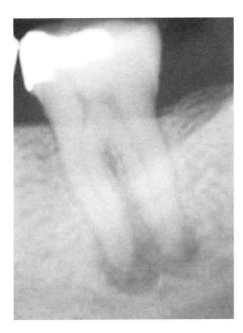

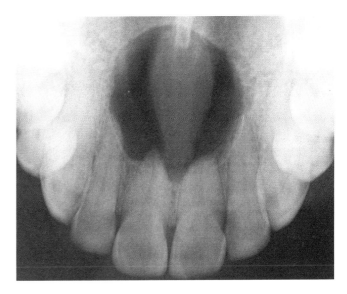

Figure 3.4 Occlusal radiograph showing a large periapical radiolucency associated with the maxillary central incisors.

Figure 3.2 Periapical radiograph showing a periapical radiolucency associated with a mandibular molar tooth.

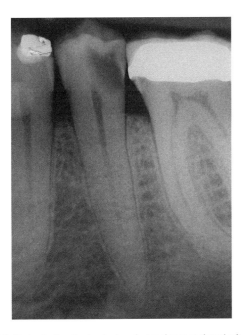

Figure 3.3 Periapical radiograph showing caries associated with a mandibular premolar tooth.

root fracture such as the unique circumferential pattern of bone loss, visible separation of the fractured fragments, or dislodgment of a root-end filling.

It must be remembered that the absence of a periapical radiolucency does not rule out the possibility of a chronic inflammatory process occurring apically. Bone loss as a consequence of an infected root canal system is detected on a radiograph only after there has been significant demineralization of the alveolar bone, usually perforation of the cortical

plate, adjacent to the apices of the affected tooth. Apart from a radiolucency, a periapical radiopacity may also be indicative of an underlying pathological process. Low-grade chronic inflammation due to an endodontic problem may cause condensing osteitis, the formation of dense, sclerotic bone around the tooth apex.

It may be necessary to take additional 'angled' views by changing the horizontal plane of the X-ray tube head by 10–15° in a distal direction to separate otherwise superimposed roots, thus allowing them to be assessed more accurately. The 'parallax principle' or 'buccal object rule' may be used to locate the relative positions, in the bucco–lingual plane, of two objects to each other, which may appear superimposed on one another. The radiographic position of the two objects will alter when the angle, either horizontal or vertical, of the X-ray tube, and therefore, the X-ray beam is changed. The more buccally located object will move in the opposite direction to which the X-ray tube is moved. Lingually or palatally located objects will move in the same direction as that of the X-ray tube. This is useful when roots overlie each other in the radiographic plane; for example, maxillary first premolars, or to distinguish between the mesial roots of a mandibular first molar.

Bitewing radiographs are a useful adjunct in those cases where the presence of proximal caries in relation to the pulp chamber anatomy needs to be confirmed. Occlusal radiographs may be used for the assessment of trauma to anterior teeth, particularly the likely presence of root fractures, and lesions that are too large to be covered on a standard periapical radiograph (Fig. 3.4). However, due the method of taking this type of radiograph, occlusal views cannot be easily reproduced, and also may result in a significant amount of distortion. A dental panoramic radiograph may also be necessary.

One of the very few indications for the use of bisecting angled radiographs is the detection of a possible horizontal root fracture. The fracture line will only be revealed if the X-ray beam passes within 15° of the plane of the fracture. Therefore, if there is a possibility of a horizontal root fracture, bisecting radiographs should be taken at two or three different horizontal angles in the same vertical plane.

Digital radiography is now becoming more common in dentistry. Instead of conventional X-ray films, two types of direct digital image receptors are available: solid state or photostimulable phosphor storage plates. The photostimulable phosphor storage plates are placed in a special processor and scanned by a laser, resulting in a digital image. The solid state sensors may be charge-coupled devices (CCD) or complementary metal oxide semiconductors (CMOS); the X-ray energy is detected and when transferred to a computer, it is processed into a digital image.

Conventional radiographic images captured on X-ray films or via digital sensors are two-dimensional 'shadowgraphs' with inherent problems of geometric distortions and anatomical noise. Recently, cone beam computed tomography (CBCT) has been introduced into dentistry. CBCT is an extraoral imaging system, which can produce

Table 3.3 Benefits of cone beam computed tomography over conventional radiography

- Three-dimensional assessment
- Accurate reproduction of structures with no distortion
- Elimination of anatomical noise

three-dimensional scans of the maxillofacial skeleton with an effective dose, which is comparable to conventional radiographs. It offers many benefits over, and can be used as an adjunct to, conventional radiography (Table 3.3). The volumetric data set obtained from the CBCT scanner is reconstructed using sophisticated computer software to allow viewing of the image in three orthogonal planes: axial, sagittal, and coronal simultaneously (Fig. 3.5). An area can be assessed by selecting and

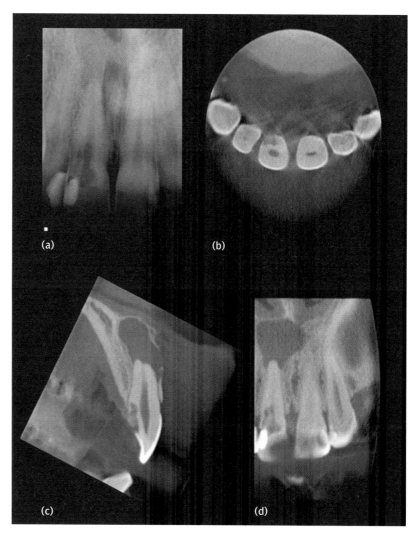

(a)

(b)

(c)

(d)

Figure 3.5 External cervical resorption: (a) conventional radiograph, and cone beam computed tomography images (b) axial, (c) sagittal, and (d) coronal planes.

moving the cursor on a chosen image, which simultaneously alters the other reconstructed slices.

In endodontics, the limited volume CBCT scans capture small volumes of data that can include just two or three individual teeth. For example, the 3D Accuitomo (J Morita Corporation, Osaka, Japan) captures a 40 mm (height) by 40 mm (diameter) volume of data, which is similar in overall height and width to a periapical radiograph. With smaller volumes, assessment and diagnosis is confined to the limited area of interest. Due to its increased sensitivity, CBCT can detect endodontic lesions which are not visible on conventional radiographs. Table 3.4 gives the indications for CBCT. It should be emphasized that the use of CBCT should be limited to complex cases that would likely be assessed and treated by a specialist in endodontics.

How do we arrive at a diagnosis?

This section covers some of the basics on how to arrive at a diagnosis and the common errors in diagnosis. The process involves collecting, assessing and interpreting all the information before arriving at a diagnosis. It is not a skill that can be learned by reading books but rather requires practice and experience. There are many, often conflicting, pieces of information that have to be assessed and prioritized. The synthesis of clinical data, higher-order thinking, critical reasoning, and problem-solving will lead to decision-making and a diagnosis, all of which takes time to learn.

Crucial to endodontic diagnosis is the relationship between symptoms, signs, and the histopathological state of the pulp. Unfortunately, these relationships are not easy to elucidate; they are not always clearly defined or reproducible. The differential diagnosis of the pulpal and periapical conditions is dependent on the presenting symptoms, clinical, and radiographic signs (Table 3.5).

As it is impossible to accurately diagnose the status of the pulp from clinical signs and symptoms, it has been argued that the descriptions: 'acute' or 'chronic' may not be appropriate. Instead, it has been suggested that the terms 'symptomatic' and 'asymptomatic' may be preferable. The terms 'apical', 'periapical' and 'periradicular' have also been used interchangeably.

Table 3.4 Indications for cone beam computed tomography in endodontics

- Identification of complex root canal anatomy, e.g. dens-in-dente, molar teeth
- Determination of the extent of a periapical radiolucency and its effect on surrounding structures
- Diagnosis and management of poorly localized orofacial pain
- Diagnosis and management of dental trauma
- Diagnosis and management of root resorption
- Treatment planning for surgical endodontics

Table 3.5 Pulpal and periapical conditions

Condition	Characteristics
Healthy pulp	Symptom-free
	Positive response to sensibility testing
Reversible pulpitis	Sharp, transient pain
	Does not linger when stimulus removed
	Often poorly localized
	No tenderness to percussion
	No obvious radiographic changes
Irreversible pulpitis	Dull, throbbing pain, may be spontaneous
	Lingers when stimulus removed
	May be kept awake at nights
	Usually no tenderness to percussion
Pulp necrosis	May or may not be painful
	No response from sensibility testing
	Usually no obvious radiographic changes
Healthy periapical tissues	No tenderness to percussion or palpation
	Lamina dura intact and uniform periodontal ligament space

Condition	Characteristics
Acute periapical periodontitis	Pain on biting and percussion or palpation
	Slightly widened periodontal ligament space
	Thinning of the lamina dura
	Periapical radiolucency may be present
Acute periapical abscess	Rapid onset, spontaneous pain
	Tooth tender to any pressure and may be mobile
	Swelling present
Chronic periapical periodontitis	Often symptom-free or only very mild symptoms
	Widened periodontal ligament space
	Periapical radiolucency present
Chronic periapical abscess	Usually symptom-free
	Sinus tract present
	Periapical radiolucency present
Condensing osteitis	Usually symptom-free
	No radiolucency, instead a periapical radiopacity

How do we take a history?

It is essential that the clinician is attentive, sympathetic, and interested in the patient's presenting complaint. This will result in the patient being more inclined to provide a full and accurate account of their complaint. It is advisable to always ask open-ended, non-leading questions instead of those that only require a 'yes' or 'no' answer. The questions asked should also be easy to understand and unbiased. By doing this, it allows the patient to explain and describe their complaint in their own words. If necessary, further questions for the purpose of clarification should be asked.

Presenting complaint

It is useful to have a mental checklist of the type of questions that should be asked that will cover the various aspects of the presenting complaint. As the majority of endodontic complaints are related to pain, the questions asked are often directed at obtaining a pain history and covering the following features:

- Character
- Duration or onset
- Periodicity
- Severity
- Site
- Radiation
- Provoking or relieving factors
- Associated factors

Therefore, the following are examples of questions that may be asked as part of endodontic history taking:

- How may I help? What is the problem?
- When did you first notice the problem? How long have you had pain?
- What does the pain feel like? How would you describe the pain?
- What brings on the pain?
- Where is the pain located?

- How long does the pain last?
- When does it hurt most?
- What makes the pain better?
- What makes the pain worse?
- Is there anything else associated with the pain?

Dental history

Examples of questions that should be asked during dental history taking include:

- Are you anxious about having dental treatment?
- Have you had any previous bad dental experiences?
- When was your last visit to a dentist or dental professional?
- How often do you attend your dentist?
- How often do you clean your teeth?
- What dental cleaning products do you use?
- Do you have a sweet tooth?
- Do you recall any trauma or knocks to your teeth?
- Have you had orthodontic treatment?
- Have you had recent dental treatment? (if so, what, where, when, and from whom?)

Medical history

A medical history questionnaire should be used to provide a comprehensive record so that no items of importance are missed. There are many examples of pro forma questionnaires, which are available from commercial sources, dental associations, or specialist societies. It is useful to ask the patient to complete the medical history questionnaire in advance and this can then be discussed during the consultation. Questions should include current and previous medications, allergies and, when appropriate, pregnancy status.

How do we carry out an extraoral examination?

An extraoral examination should be carried out by viewing the patient from the front and also from above and from the back while they are in a reclined position in the dental chair. The extraoral examination should include assessment of:

- Patient cooperation: can the patient tolerate treatment in a supine position?
- Facial asymmetry;

- Extraoral swelling, including size, location, consistency;
- Extraoral sinus tracts (Fig. 3.6);
- Trauma to the orofacial region;
- Head and neck lymph nodes for lymphadenopathy;
- Temporomandibular joint dysfunction, e.g. tenderness to palpation of the muscles of mastication, clicking or crepitus of the temporomandibular joint.

How do we carry out an intraoral examination?

Magnification, e.g. dental loupes or dental operating microscope, and coaxial illumination are helpful for carrying out an intraoral examination. The intraoral examination should include assessment of:

- Patient's tolerance of dentistry;
- General examination of the mouth;
- Specific examination of the area(s) of main complaint.

Patient's tolerance of dentistry

Patient's tolerance of dentistry should be assessed, including:

- Mouth opening (Fig. 3.7). Does the patient have adequate mouth opening to access the tooth? Can the patient open their mouth adequately and comfortably for a long period of time?

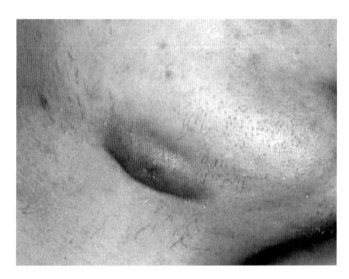

Figure 3.6 Extraoral sinus tract.

- Gag reflex. Can the patient tolerate radiographs and rubber dam?

It may be challenging to perform endodontic treatment if the patient has restricted mouth opening or a strong gag reflex.

General examination of the mouth

The general state of the oral cavity should be surveyed before homing in on the area of interest related to the main complaint. The general examination should include checking for the following:

- Abnormal appearance of the oral mucosa, e.g. sinus tract, ulceration or erythema;
- Frictional keratosis or scalloping of the tongue (common signs of parafunction);
- Presence, location, tenderness, consistency, and size of any soft tissue abnormalities and swellings;
- Missing or unopposed teeth;
- Oral hygiene status (Fig. 3.8) and basic periodontal examination;
- Food traps (Fig. 3.9) and plaque-retentive factors;
- Tooth discolouration (Fig. 3.1);
- Tooth surface loss (Fig. 3.10);
- Caries (Fig 3.11);
- Quality and quantity of the existing dental treatment or restorations (Fig 3.12);
- Signs of marginal leakage (Fig. 3.12);
- Fractured teeth or restorations (Fig. 3.13).

All of this information should then be correlated to the patient's past dental history.

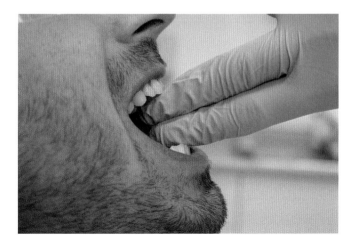

Figure 3.7 The extent of mouth opening and access for treatment gauged using fingers of a gloved hand.

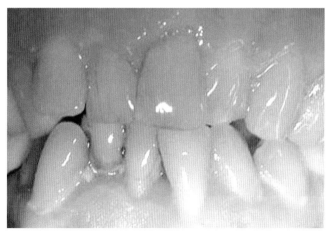

Figure 3.8 Patient with poor oral hygiene; note plaque accumulation at the gingival margins of the anterior teeth.

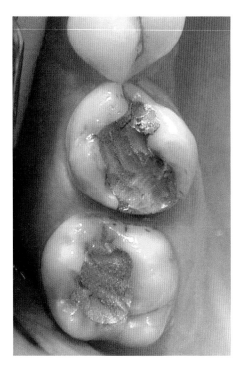

Figure 3.9 Open contact between the maxillary first and second molar teeth may result in food packing interproximally.

Specific examination of the area(s) of main complaint

The area(s) in question should be assessed visually in the first instance. The location, size, and consistency, e.g. rubbery, firm, or fluctuant and localized or diffused, of any soft or hard tissue swellings should be noted

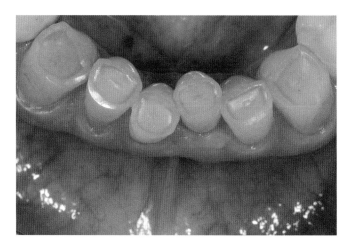

Figure 3.10 Marked tooth surface loss may affect the integrity of the pulp.

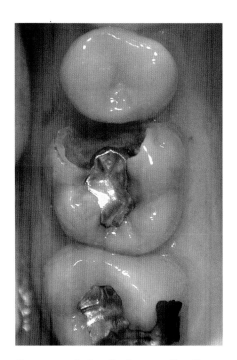

Figure 3.11 Caries affecting a maxillary first molar tooth.

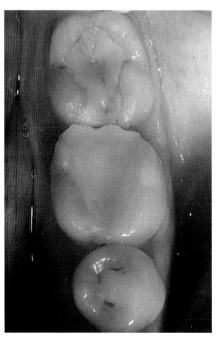

Figure 3.12 Unsatisfactory contact between the restorations in the mandibular first and second molar teeth. There are also signs of marginal leakage with the restoration in the mandibular second molar tooth.

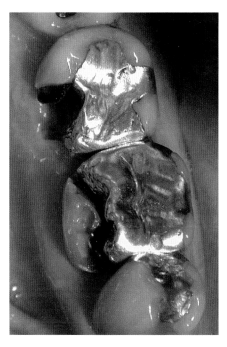

Figure 3.13 Fractured teeth and restorations.

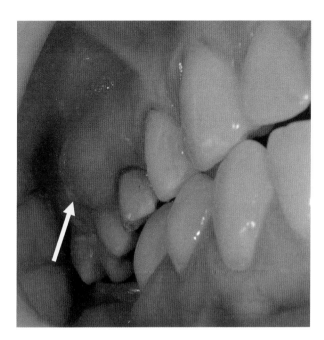

Figure 3.14 Intraoral swelling (yellow arrow) related to a maxillary posterior tooth.

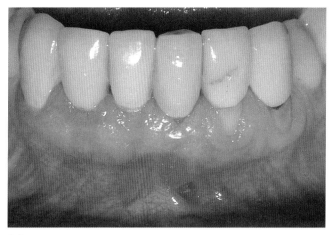

(a)

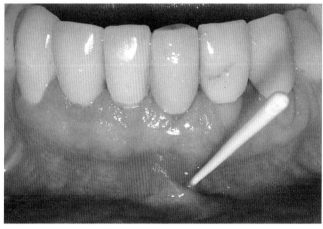

(b)

Figure 3.15 (a) Careful assessment of the soft tissues is essential; a Labial sinus tract associated with mandibular incisor teeth. (b) GP point in sinus tract in preparation for a periapical radiograph to be taken.

(Fig. 3.14). Similarly, any abnormal appearance of the mucosa overlying the area in question, for example, the presence of a sinus tract (Fig. 3.15a) should be noted. If a sinus tract is present, its origin may be traced with a gutta-percha (GP) point (Fig. 3.15b) and then taking a radiograph. Where appropriate, diagrams, and photographs of the relevant findings may be used to supplement note-taking.

The next stage is to carry out the following: assessment of the periodontal condition of the tooth or teeth in question.

Palpation

The mucosa on either side of the area related to the main complaint should be palpated gently using finger pressure (Fig. 3.16). A note should be made of any tenderness, the extent and severity; the contralateral and adjacent quadrant should also be palpated for comparison. Tenderness or swelling of the overlying mucosa usually indicates that infection or inflammation has extended beyond the apex and into the overlying soft tissues.

Percussion

The tooth or teeth should, initially, be gently pressed with a finger to see if there is any tenderness. If necessary, greater force may be applied using the end of a mirror handle (Fig. 3.17). However, the end of a mirror handle should never be used with unnecessary force when carrying out this test. With a posterior tooth, it is important to tap each cusp and therefore, each root, as only one root may be tender to percussion. Tenderness to percussion indicates that infection or inflammation has involved the periodontal ligament. However, a common non-endodontic cause is occlusal trauma from bruxism.

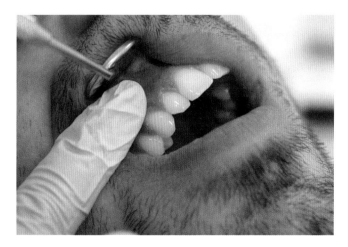

Figure 3.16 Tenderness to palpation assessed by gently pressing the mucosa.

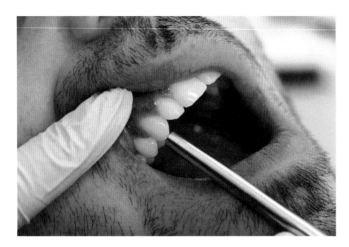

Figure 3.17 Gentle percussion of a tooth with a mirror handle.

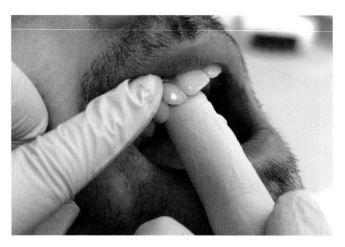

Figure 3.18 Mobility assessed by applying fingertip pressure to the opposing sides of the tooth.

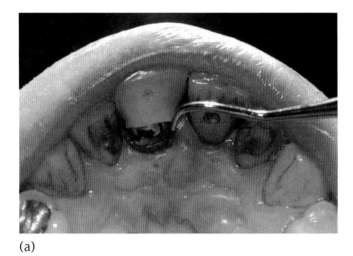

(a)

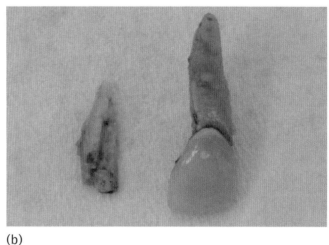

(b)

Figure 3.19 Vertical root fracture of a maxillary central incisor restored with a post-retained crown. (a) 'Walking' the periodontal probe around the gingival sulcus reveals a deep, isolated, and narrow periodontal pocket adjacent to the fracture line. (b) Fractured tooth fragments following extraction.

Mobility

Tooth mobility should be noted and graded according to the extent. Excessive mobility may be due to loss of attachment as a result of chronic periodontal disease or an acutely inflamed periodontal ligament resulting from pulpitis or occlusal trauma. Other common causes of excessive mobility include a vertical or horizontal root fracture or a decemented post.

With fingers (Fig. 3.18) or the end of two mirror handles placed on opposing sides of the tooth, pressure is applied in both vertical and horizontal directions. The extent of any mobility is graded accordingly:

- Grade I: just perceptible, slightly more than normal movement;
- Grade II: >1 mm in any horizontal direction;
- Grade III: >1 mm in any horizontal or vertical directions.

Periodontal probing

A detailed periodontal examination should be carried out on the tooth under investigation. Attachment loss may be due to periodontal disease, vertical root fracture, or iatrogenically-induced perforation. When carrying out periodontal probing (Fig. 3.19a), the periodontal probe should be 'walked' around the whole circumference of the tooth. Otherwise, it is not uncommon to miss an isolated pocket, which may be indicative of a vertical root fracture (Fig. 3.19b).

Occlusal examination

Occlusal examination comprises:

- Assessing for signs of excess occlusal loading or trauma, and parafunctional habits (clenching and/or grinding).
- Assessing the occlusion in retruded contact and intercuspal positions, and then lateral excursions. Articulating paper may be used to identify points of premature contact.

Occlusal factors may cause:

- Temporomandibular joint or related muscle pain, which may present as symptoms similar to pulpal or periapical disease.
- Propagation of cracks in teeth, which may then give rise to endodontic problems, such as 'cracked tooth syndrome' or, by acting as an entry route for microbes leading to pulpal inflammation, necrosis and infection.

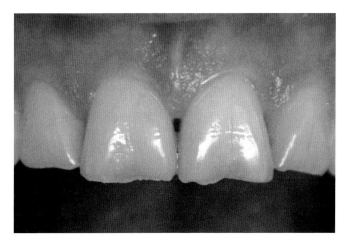

Figure 3.20 Enamel infraction lines associated with maxillary incisor teeth.

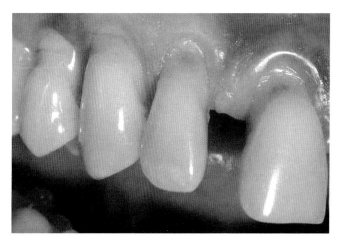

Figure 3.22 Exposed cervical dentine.

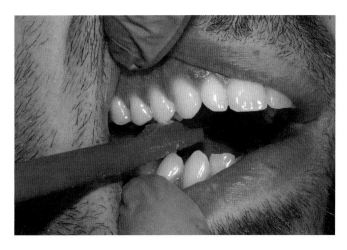

Figure 3.21 The 'wedge test'. This consists of placing a wedging device in the form of a 'tooth slooth' over a selected cusp and then asking the patient to close down firmly. If a crack is present, then the wedging forces will provoke a painful response.

Assessment of teeth

The strategic nature of the tooth or teeth under investigation should be assessed as this may well have a bearing on the final treatment plan. For example, an unopposed and non-functional tooth may be better extracted.

A note should be made of any breach of tooth structure, as this may initiate and perpetuate pulpal and periapical diseases. Magnification in the form of dental loupes or operating microscope is of tremendous help. It is important to look out for:

- Infractions, crazing, and fracture lines in the enamel (Fig. 3.20). Detection may be aided by transillumination, special dyes or a tooth slooth (Fig. 3.21).
- Primary and recurrent secondary caries (Fig. 3.11).
- Restorations with signs of microleakage or macroleakage (Fig. 3.12); for example, ditching, open, and discoloured margins, which causes plaque retention, may lead to pulpal involvement, or food packing, which may mimic pulpal symptoms.
- Exposed dentine may give rise to thermal hypersensitivity or pulpal changes (Fig. 3.22).
- Exposed pulpal tissues, for example, a complete crown fracture following trauma, or gross caries.

An assessment should be made as to the likely amount of sound coronal tooth tissue that would remain after removal of caries and the previous restorations as this will provide guidance as to the restorability of the tooth. Endodontic treatment is futile when carried out on a tooth that is clearly unrestorable. It is also pertinent to consider the type of post-endodontic restoration the tooth may require as part of treatment planning.

Any colour differences should be noted (Fig. 3.1) as these may be a sign of pulpal haemorrhage, pulpal necrosis, microleakage, or staining from the root canal filling material. The following should be recorded:

- Intrinsic or extrinsic discolouration;
- Degree of discolouration;
- Uniformity of the discolouration;
- Extent of the discolouration, i.e. partial or total.

How do we carry out special investigations?

Sensibility testing

The following are essential for predictable and accurate sensibility testing:

- Explain and advise patient of the test;
- Request that the patient indicate, for example, by raising a hand when the stimulus is felt;

- Dry the tooth to be tested with gauze or cotton wool pledgets;
- Isolate the tooth with cotton wool rolls;
- As a control, test a healthy tooth first;
- Test the questionable tooth next;
- Test an adjacent and a contralateral tooth to gain a more objective comparison;

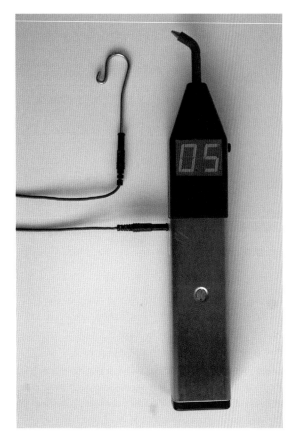

Figure 3.23 An electric pulp tester: Digitest (Parkell, Edgewood, NY, USA).

- Test both the buccal and lingual or palatal aspects of multirooted teeth;
- Repeat the test if necessary;
- Be aware of false positive or false negative test results;
- Record all the findings.

Electric testing

An electric current from a battery-operated device (Fig. 3.23) is used as the stimulus in this test. A small clip is hooked onto the patient's lip and the probe is placed on the coronal half, usually the buccal surface (Fig. 3.24), of the tooth in question to complete the circuit. Alternatively, the patient is allowed to hold the handle of the test probe, which is in contact with the tooth and this completes the circuit. A conducting medium such as toothpaste or prophylaxis paste is essential to improve the conduction of the electrical current from the probe to the tooth. The patient is asked to indicate by, for example, raising a hand, or letting go if they are holding the handle of the test probe, when they feel warmth or tingling on the tooth being tested. With most of the electric pulp testers on the market, the electric current passing through the tooth will increase automatically the longer the probe is in contact with the tooth; the rate at which the current increases may also be adjusted. If a tooth has a full coronal coverage restoration, e.g. a crown, there is no natural

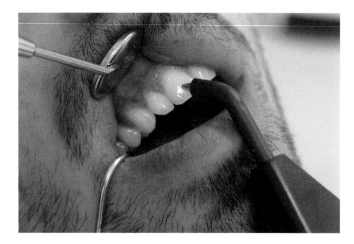

Figure 3.24 An electric pulp tester in use. The probe of the electric pulp tester is placed on the buccal surface of the tooth. Note the lip clip resting on the corner of the mouth to complete the circuit.

tooth surface for probe placement to carry out electric pulp testing. With some electric pulp testers, a finer probe is available and it may just be possible to place this fine probe on uncovered tooth tissue near the crown margins.

Cold testing

Cold tests can be performed using a variety of materials and equipment:

- Ice;
- Ice cold water while the tooth is isolated under rubber dam;
- Ice crystals formed on foam pellets or cotton wool pledgets using ethyl chloride or refrigerant sprays;
- Dry ice sticks (CO_2 snow).

It is generally accepted that the colder the stimulus, the more reliable the test. Ice and ethyl chloride are not cold enough to be sufficiently discriminatory and may give rise to false negative results. Refrigerant spray is recommended as it is easy to use and also readily available. This is applied to a foam pellet or cotton wool pledget. Sufficient time should be allowed for ice crystals to form prior to application on the tooth surface (Fig. 3.25).

Heat testing

Heat tests can be performed using a variety of materials and equipment:

- Warm GP point/pellet/stick (Fig. 3.26a). The point of application on the tooth should first be coated with a separating medium, such as petroleum jelly, to prevent the warm GP from sticking to the tooth;
- Warm, not hot or boiling, water while the tooth is isolated under rubber dam (Fig. 3.26b);
- Heated probe, e.g. Elements Obturation Unit (SybronEndo, Orange, CA, USA);
- A rotating prophy cup to create frictional heat.

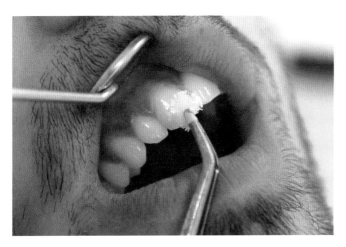

Figure 3.25 Cold testing being carried out; ice crystals have formed on the foam pellet following application of a refrigerant spray.

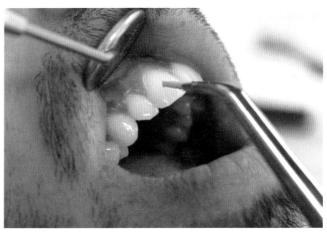

(a)

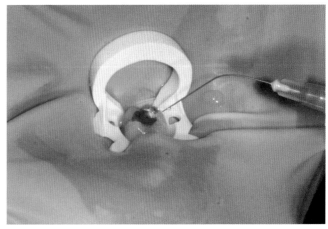

(b)

Figure 3.26 Heat testing being carried out: (a) using a warm GP point and (b) by applying syringed warm water on to a tooth isolated with rubber dam.

Test cavity preparation

As a last resort, a small test cavity may be prepared in the tooth but without local anaesthetic. The patient is advised to signal if any pain is felt. It is prudent to be aware that with some patients, especially if they are nervous, a false positive result may be obtained. It must be emphasized that indiscriminate test cavity preparation purely for the purpose of ascertaining pulpal health is inadvisable.

Radiographic examination

Every aspect of endodontics is heavily reliant upon information gained from radiography. Radiographs are usually needed preoperatively, during treatment, postoperatively, and at reviews.

Periapical radiographs

Radiographs (film-based or digital) should be taken using a beam-aiming, paralleling device to ensure undistorted and reproducible images (Fig. 3.27a,b,c,d). These devices are designed for use with both anterior and posterior teeth. The radiograph should show the whole tooth together with at least 3–4 mm of surrounding bone (Fig. 3.28a,b). When examining a periapical radiograph, start initially with an overview of the teeth and structures visible. Next, focus on the area of interest and then the tooth or teeth concerned. The features to note and to assess when viewing a periapical radiograph are covered in Table 3.6. If there is an intraoral or extraoral sinus, the source of the infection may be traced by

inserting a GP point into the sinus tract (Fig. 3.29a) and taking a periapical radiograph (Fig. 3.29b).

Parallax views

This involves taking two periapical radiographs at slightly different horizontal angles of about 10–15 degrees (Fig. 3.30a,b). A horizontal shift of the X-ray tube may produce more relevant information about the tooth under investigation (Fig. 3.31a,b).

What are the common errors in diagnosis?

Endodontic diseases usually manifest clinically in the form of pain, swelling, and/or a periapical radiolucency. However, the clinician should always be aware that there are also non-endodontic causes, which may mimic endodontic problems; detailed explanations on the subject are provided in standard texts on oral medicine and oral pathology and they should be consulted.

Radiographic errors

In a symptom-free situation, the only sign of endodontic disease may be a periapical radiolucency and this may be an incidental radiographic finding. For example, an infected necrotic root canal system associated with chronic apical periodontitis (Fig. 3.32). However, it should be

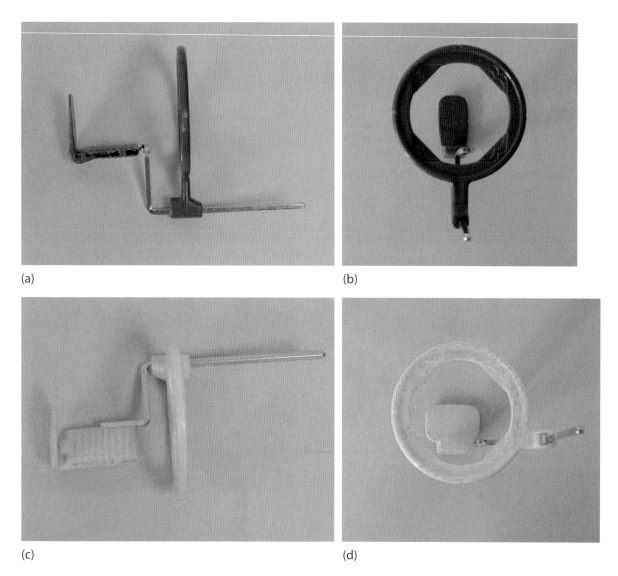

(a)　　　　　　　　　　　　　　(b)

(c)　　　　　　　　　　　　　　(d)

Figure 3.27 Beam-aiming paralleling devices: (a,b) for anterior teeth and (c,d) for posterior teeth.

remembered that not all radiolucencies are indicative of pathosis. For example, the radiographic appearance of the mental foramen may be mistaken for a lesion (Fig. 3.33).

Alternatively, radiographic examination may reveal a radiographic lesion not related to the patient's perceived problems but in the region of the reported problem area; this may be attributed wrongly to the symptoms or clinical findings. It may result in misdiagnosis and, possibly, the wrong treatment being carried out.

A differential diagnosis of radiographic lesions is dependent on the location, size, shape, radiodensity, outline, and effect on neighbouring structures. A summary is shown in Table 3.7. and revision on the subject by consulting the relevant books is recommended. Examples of errors that occur when over-reliance is placed on radiographic findings alone include the following:

Anatomical landmarks

The radiolucent shadows of the mental and incisive foramina may be mistaken for lesions associated with pulpal or periapical diseases. Sensibility testing will help confirm that these 'radiolucencies' are anatomical landmarks. Additional existing radiographs, for example panoramic views, showing the contralateral side may also help confirm the position of the mental foramen, which should be in a symmetrically similar location. Widening of the periodontal ligament space and apparent radiolucencies may also be due to superimposition of root apices over the maxillary sinuses and the inferior dental canal. Sparse bony trabeculation and varying bone density may also be mistaken for pathosis.

Periapical osseous dysplasia

A condition, also known as periapical fibro-cemento-osseous dysplasia, in which bone is replaced by fibrous tissue, which is then replaced with bone or mineralized tissue to varying degrees. The lesions are usually associated with the apices of mandibular incisor teeth and may be mistaken for periapical lesions. Sensibility testing and even follow-up radiographs will help confirm that there is no pathosis.

Non-inflammatory swellings

Although non-inflammatory swellings have unique presenting features, in reality, the range of presenting features does not preclude their occasional

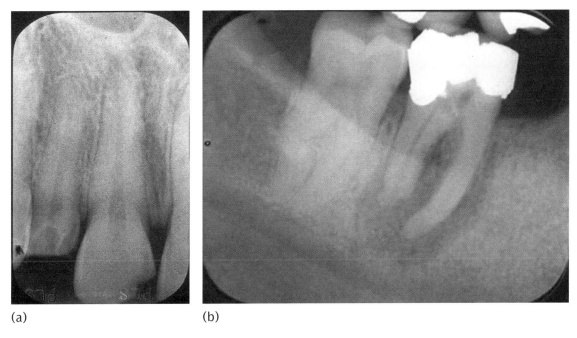

Figure 3.28 Periapical radiographs taken using a beam-aiming paralleling device: (a) anterior and (b) posterior.

Table 3.6 Radiographic features to note and to assess when viewing a periapical radiograph

General overview	Tooth and area of interest
Note:	— Continuity and width of the periodontal ligament space
• Caries	— Integrity and thickness of the lamina dura
• Periodontal health	— Presence of any radiolucent or radiopaque areas
• State of existing restoration	• Roots and root canal system
• Quality of any previous root fillings	— Number of roots
• Evidence of any abnormalities/pathosis	— Length of roots
Tooth and area of interest	— Root morphology and curvatures
Assess:	— Root canal outline
• Crown of tooth	— Root resorption
— Caries	— Root fracture
— State of existing restoration	— Root canal or pulp chamber calcifications
— Amount of tooth structure	— Quality and type of any root canal fillings present
• Periodontal and periapical tissues	— Iatrogenic problems e.g. separated file, root perforation
— Level and quality of crestal bone	
— Vertical/horizontal/furcation bone loss	

and passing resemblance to those of periapical origin. It is important to be familiar with the characteristics of these conditions and be able to differentiate between them. Details of such diseases are covered comprehensively in more appropriate texts; a summary is provided in Table 3.7.

Treatment planning

Once a diagnosis has been reached, the patient should be advised of the various treatment options available. For each treatment option, the patient should be advised of the following:

• Advantages and disadvantages;

• Prognosis or expected treatment outcome;

• Time involved and number of appointments needed;

• Cost implications if applicable;

• Risks and possible complications.

The patient can only make an informed decision on the most suitable treatment once each option has been discussed (see Chapter 10). The principle of informed consent requires that the patient is advised on the most appropriate treatment option after all options have been explained.

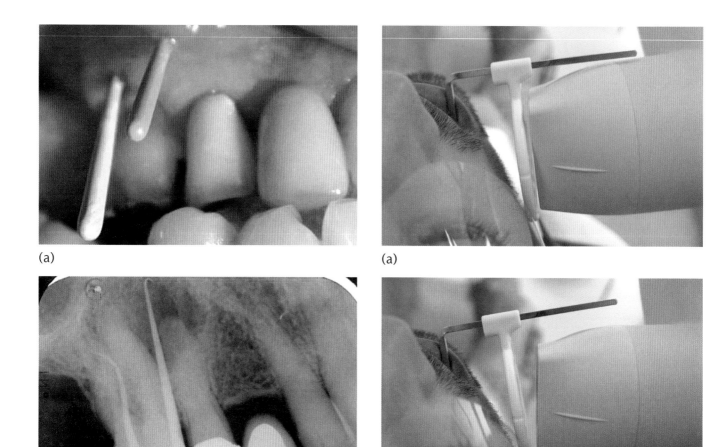

Figure 3.29 Two GP points have been used to 'track' the sinus tracts: (a) clinical view and (b) periapical radiograph.

Figure 3.30 Parallax radiography: two periapical radiographs are taken (a) straight on and (b) with a horizontal shift of 10 degrees to the distal.

What is a treatment plan?

A treatment plan is a list of procedures, a timetable, individually tailored for each patient, based on their unique dental problem(s) and needs. The treatment plan aims to address patient care in an ordered, systematic, and logical fashion. It can be broken down into different phases:

• Pain relief;

• Disease stabilization including oral hygiene instruction and dietary advice;

• Maintaining or restoring function;

• Maintaining or restoring aesthetics;

• Review or maintenance.

A treatment plan may be relatively simple if there is only a single, solitary problem in need of attention. In other cases, it may be more complicated, requiring a multidisciplinary approach that needs to be broken down into phases of implementation such as those mentioned above. The initial treatment plan may also have to be modified, to allow for unplanned or unforeseen circumstances along the way. An example of this is where

root canal treatment has been planned but upon accessing the tooth or removing the existing restoration, a vertical fracture is detected (Fig. 3.34). If a fracture such as this runs through the pulp chamber, mesio-distally, the tooth is split and untreatable. The treatment plan would obviously need to be modified as the tooth would need to be extracted and other treatment options for the resultant space discussed.

Where does endodontic treatment fit in treatment planning?

Initial phase

The initial phase is usually to relieve pain by, for example, pulp extirpation or incision and drainage.

Definitive phase

The definitive phase is disease stabilization. The aim is to eliminate dental disease and its aetiological factors, e.g. caries stabilization or root canal treatment and replacement of leaking restorations with well-adapted ones. Once root canal treatment has been completed, the tooth

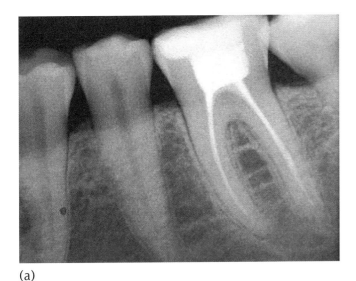

(a)

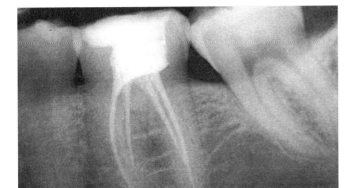

(b)

Figure 3.31 Parallax views of an endodontically treated mandibular molar tooth provide a better appreciation of the quality of the root canal fillings in both the mesial and distal roots: (a) normal view and (b) distal view.

should be permanently restored so that it may be rendered functional again (see Chapter 7).

Maintenance and review

It is important to assess the outcome of endodontic treatment (see Chapter 8). Follow-up may reveal that treatment has an unfavourable outcome and this may mean that retreatment or extraction may be required.

Record keeping

It is imperative to keep good and comprehensive records, including noting down all discussions about treatment options and plans. Dento-legally, it should be remembered that 'no records equals no defence' should there be any potential misunderstanding or future litigation (see Chapter 10). In addition, before starting any treatment, consent must be obtained and this it must be recorded.

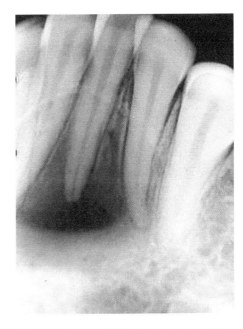

Figure 3.32 Large periapical radiolucency associated with symptom-free teeth.

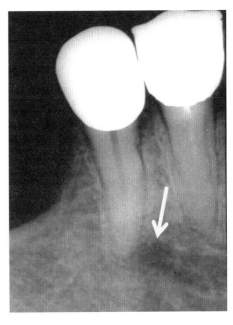

Figure 3.33 Radiographic appearance of the mental foramen (yellow arrow) may be mistaken for the presence of apical pathosis.

What are the factors that influence treatment planning?

Patient-related factors

These factors include the patient's medical and dental history, expectations, motivation, attitude, and compliance with treatment. Occasionally, a patient's expectations may be unrealistic or more importantly focus on other perceived problems that may not be immediately obvious or important. Unless the patient is cooperative it would be challenging trying to carry out the treatment plan.

Table 3.7 Differential diagnosis of radiolucent lesions and swellings

Radiolucent lesions

- Normal anatomy, e.g. mental foramen
- Artefacts, e.g. processing errors
- Pathological
  - Infection
  - Trauma
  - Cyst
  - Tumour or tumour-like lesion
  - Giant cell lesion
  - Fibro-cemento-osseous lesion

Swellings

- Abscess of dental origin
- Cysts (odontogenic more common than non-odontogenic)
- Odontogenic tumours
- Giant cell lesions
- Fibro-osseous lesions
- Non-odontogenic neoplasms of bone

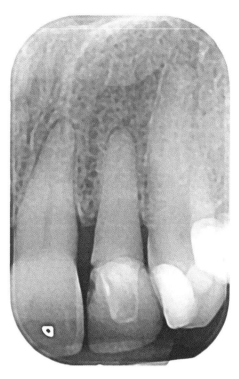

Figure 3.35 Calcified root canal associated with a maxillary lateral incisor tooth.

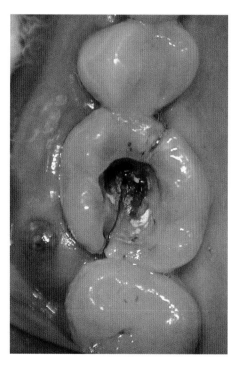

Figure 3.34 Fracture running mesio-distally through a maxillary first molar tooth.

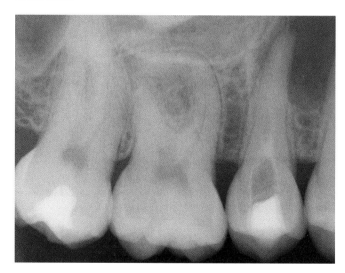

Figure 3.36 Acute curvature associated with the mesio-buccal root of a maxillary first molar tooth.

Dental-related factors

As mentioned previously, the dental factors that may influence treatment planning include:

- Access;
- Oral hygiene standard;
- Periodontal support;
- Importance and strategic nature of the tooth;
- Restorability.

In terms of dental anatomy, endodontic management may be influenced by:

- Size of the pulp chamber and presence of any calcifications;
- Number of root canals and their relative size and degree of any calcification (Fig. 3.35);
- Complexity of root canal contour and curvature (Fig. 3.36);

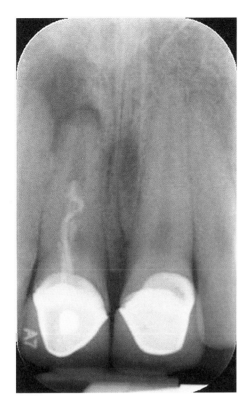

Figure 3.37 An under-extended and poorly compacted root canal filling associated with a maxillary central incisor tooth.

- If a tooth has already been endodontically treated, the quality of the root canal filling (Fig. 3.37) and the presence of foreign objects such as a separated instrument.

Clinician-related factors

Knowledge, experience, and the skill of the clinician are all important considerations in treatment planning. These factors will influence the treatment options the clinician is able to offer to the patient and will impact on the decision-making process. Access to equipment (e.g.

dental operating microscope) and secondary dental care (e.g specialist in endodontics) may also influence the treatment approach adopted.

Complex problems and challenging cases are often best managed by specialists in endodontics. Regulatory bodies and dento-legal defence organizations have also advised that, where necessary, patients should be referred for further advice or treatment, or if requested by the patient.

Various specialist societies and organizations have developed endodontic case assessment forms. For example, the American Association of Endodontists' Endodontic Case Difficulty Assessment Form, is intended to assist clinicians with endodontic treatment planning. The assessment form identifies areas requiring consideration, which may affect treatment complexity, e.g. patient considerations, diagnostic, and treatment considerations, and other additional considerations. Within each category, levels of difficulty are assigned based upon potential risk factors. Depending on the level of difficulty in an individual case, the clinician can then decide whether to undertake the treatment or to refer the case to a specialist.

What does decision-making involve?

Decision-making involves analysis of all the elicited information, prioritizing, and 'weighing up' all the pieces of information, and giving balanced consideration to the various factors involved. Clinicians are challenged by the need for accountability. Fundamental to accountability are the concepts of risk assessment and evidence-based practice. Risk assessment is the formal procedure of evaluating the significance of risks in order to facilitate the decision-making process. Case difficulty assessment tools such as that mentioned earlier may be used. As for evidence-based practice, it requires the conscientious, explicit, and judicious use of current best evidence for the care of individual patients.

With growing knowledge, confidence, and experience, the process of decision-making and the formulation of treatment plans will gradually become easier and more routine. Whilst a novice may find the decision-making process slow and frustrating, a step-by-step approach is essential to the development of competence and, ultimately, expertise.

Patient management

The remainder of this chapter is a brief summary of the issues that may be pertinent to patient management if endodontic treatment is provided. It is not meant to be comprehensive but based on commonly encountered clinical scenarios.

Local anaesthesia

Good and adequate anaesthesia is essential for endodontic treatment, to ensure the patient is comfortable, and to maintain the patient's confidence and trust. A significant number of patients are very nervous of dental treatment; they may have had painful treatment experiences in the past or may already be in considerable pain. The fear of pain itself may often be the reason why some patients defer or do not seek treatment.

To try and ensure that successful and adequate local anaesthesia is achieved:

- Decide on the appropriate local anaesthetic technique;
- Choose the most suitable type of local anaesthetic solution;
- Apply topical anaesthetic to the injection site if applicable;
- Administer injections slowly using a self-aspirating syringe;
- Ensure that an adequate volume of local anaesthetic is administered;
- Confirm good anaesthesia has been achieved before starting treatment by, for example, gently probing the mucosa in the area that has been anaesthetized;
- Advise patient to indicate, for example, raising a hand if they feel any pain or discomfort;
- Advise the patient that it is normal to feel some pressure and vibration;
- Begin treatment only when anaesthesia has been successful achieved.

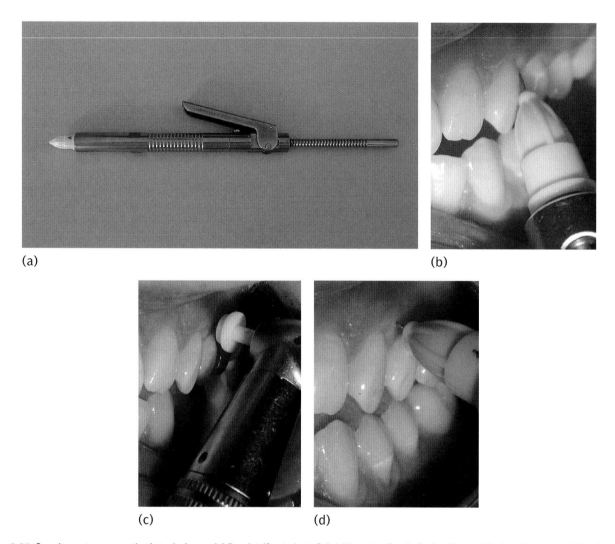

(a)

(b)

(c)   (d)

Figure 3.38 Supplementary anaesthetic techniques: (a) Parojet (Septodont, Saint-Maur-des-fossés Cedex, France) for intraligamental injection; (b) the needle placed along the long axis of the root for the intraligamental injection; (c) intraosseous e.g. Stabident system (Fairfax Dental Inc., Miami, FL, USA), a slow-speed contra-angle handpiece with a perforator penetrating the buccal cortical plate); (d) the needle (identical gauge to perforator) is introduced into the drilled hole created by perforator and the local anaesthetic delivered.

Many factors may influence the effectiveness of local anaesthesia including the choice of anaesthetic drug, its mechanism of action, the methods of administration; there are also factors that may modulate their effectiveness. For maxillary teeth, an infiltration technique into the buccal mucosa adjacent to the roots of the tooth to be treated may be adequate. However, it is advisable to consider supplementing the customary buccal infiltration with a palatal infiltration of local anaesthetic.

Infiltration techniques to anaesthetize premolar and molar teeth are rarely successful in the mandible due to the thickness of the cortical bone. It is advisable to use an inferior dental nerve block, which may be supplemented with the mental nerve block for lower anterior teeth. The inferior dental nerve block may also be supplemented with injections to anaesthetize the long buccal nerve.

If these are not successful, additional or supplementary anaesthetic techniques (Fig. 3.38) may be required including:

- Regional nerve blocks, e.g. for maxillary teeth;
- Intraligamental (Fig. 3.38a,b);
- Intraosseous (Fig. 3.38c,d);
- Intrapulpal;
- Alternative techniques, e.g. Gow-Gates or Akinosi for the inferior dental nerve.

For further information, books on local anaesthesia in dentistry should be consulted.

In extreme circumstances, despite the use of a variety of local anaesthetic techniques, it may still not be possible to achieve adequate anaesthesia. Reasons for failure of anaesthesia include:

- Poor technique;
- Inadequate amounts of local anaesthetic administered;
- Variation in patient's anatomy;
- Very inflamed tissues;
- Variation in absorption, metabolism, and excretion of local anaesthetic drug;
- Psychological factors.

In these cases, some form of sedation, whether oral or intravenous, may have to be considered. Again, this subject is best covered in the relevant textbooks.

Patients may still be in some discomfort after treatment has been completed, especially if they have been experiencing pain beforehand. They should be given reassurance and advised that it is normal to be in some discomfort for several days after treatment. Therefore, they should be given pain relief advice including continuing with any analgesics they may have been taking. A courtesy telephone call one or two days later to enquire about a patient's well-being is also recommended, as it is of tremendous psychological benefit.

Non-steroidal anti-inflammatory drugs (NSAID), such as ibuprofen, is the first drug of choice for post-operative pain. If not completely effective it may be supplemented with paracetamol (acetoaminophen) or codeine phosphate/paracetamol preparations. Whichever analgesic is chosen, it is imperative to ensure that it is tolerated by the patient and does not interfere with any medication the patient may be taking. Very rarely, a stronger opioid-based analgesic may have to be prescribed if pain relief from over-the-counter analgesics is insufficient or ineffective.

Vital pulp extirpation

Extirpation is indicated when the pulp is irreversibly inflamed. Profound anaesthesia is required for successful extirpation. Unfortunately, it is sometimes difficult to achieve good anaesthesia with a 'hot tooth' due to the extent of the inflammation. Supplemental anaesthetic techniques may be required and it is essential to advise patients, especially if they are nervous, that they may feel some discomfort or pain during the procedure.

Incision and drainage

A localized swelling, either intraoral or extraoral, must be treated as a matter of urgency. In extreme cases the swelling may result in life-threatening conditions, for example Ludwig's angina or septicaemia. An attempt must be made to incise and drain the swelling, especially if it is fluctuant. Adequate drainage will result in immediate pain relief and a reduction in the size of the swelling.

Administration of local anaesthetic directly into the affected area is often contraindicated in these situations as it may help spread the infection along the fascial planes and the anaesthetic solution may not be very effective because of the acute inflammation. Where possible, regional or nerve block type anaesthetic are more appropriate. Otherwise, limited surface anaesthesia may be achieved using a topical anaesthetic or ethyl chloride.

To incise and drain an intraoral swelling:

- Explain to the patient the incision and drainage procedure;
- Palpate the swelling gently to confirm that it is fluctuant;
- Lance the area, in one quick stroke, with the tip of scalpel blade;
- Gently massage either side of swelling with fingers to express as much pus as possible;
- Aspirate the discharge and wait until the exudation to cease;
- Give supportive care advice, e.g. analgesics, plenty of fluids and a soft diet.

In addition to incision and drainage of any intraoral fluctuant swelling, drainage via the root canal system (Fig. 3.39) should also be attempted.

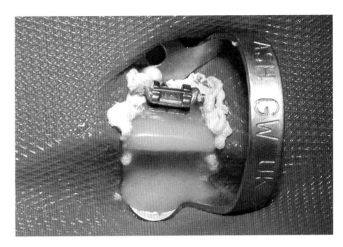

Figure 3.39 Drainage of pus obtained through the root canal. A caulking agent was necessary to seal the margins of the rubber dam.

To achieve successful drainage via the root canal system:

- Explain the proposed procedure to the patient;
- Support the tooth with, for example, a finger to reduce the vibration from the handpiece;
- Gain access into the root canal(s);
- If necessary, explore the root canal(s) with a fine file to facilitate drainage;
- Gently massage the associated swelling with fingers to express as much pus as possible though the root canal(s);
- Once drainage from the root canal(s) has stopped, irrigate the pulp space copiously;
- Medicate the tooth and place a temporary filling;
- If extruded from the socket, adjust the tooth so that it is out of occlusion;
- Prescribe antibiotics if there are signs of systemic involvement;
- Give supportive care advice, e.g. analgesics, plenty of fluids and soft diet.

The routine practice of gaining access and leaving the tooth opened to drain is to be discouraged. If left opened, over time, it will allow the entry of oral microbes, foreign objects, and food debris into the root canal system further complicating endodontic management.

Antibiotics

Antibiotics should not be prescribed as the first line of treatment for dentoalveolar abscesses. If prescribed, antibiotics are only an adjunct to treatment. They do not actually treat abscesses or their cause(s); they are used to limit swelling and to prevent spread of the infection. The overzealous use of antibiotics as a 'quick fix' is to be discouraged as it is not a long-term solution and it may also result in microbes developing increased resistance to antibiotics.

The majority of dentoalveolar abscesses can be treated without antibiotics but there are situations where they are indicated. For example, if a patient presents with a diffused swelling that cannot be

Table 3.8 Suggested regimes for adult patients requiring antibiotics

Amoxicillin	By mouth, 250–500 mg every 8 hours for 5 days
and/or	
Metronidazole	By mouth, 200–400 mg every 8 hours for 5 days, *no alcohol*
If allergic to penicillin:	
Clindamycin	By mouth, 150–300 mg every 6 hours for 5 days
or	
Erythromycin	By mouth, 250–500 mg every 6 hours for 5 days

adequately drained via the root canal system or by incision and drainage. If the infection is spreading, invading the fascial spaces below the mandible or the orbital area. If there is cervical lympadenopathy and a raised temperature, usually in association with malaise, which are indications of systemic spread of infection, antibiotics should be prescribed.

When prescribing a course of antibiotics, the following should be considered:

- Signs of systemic involvement ;
- Antibiotics would not interfere with other medications or existing medical conditions;
- The most suitable antibiotic, an adequate dose, duration, and suitable route of administration;
- The patient is advised of any possible interactions or side-effects.

Commonly suggested antibiotics and regimes are shown in Table 3.8.

Preparatory treatment of a broken-down tooth prior to endodontic treatment

It is not uncommon that a broken down or grossly carious tooth may not be easy to isolate with rubber dam. The disassembly of a complex restoration may also mean that there is limited coronal tooth structure to provide rubber dam retention. In these cases, it is strongly advisable to build up a provisional core or temporary restoration prior to starting endodontic treatment.

The core may be placed with the aid of a matrix band, a suitably trimmed copper band, or orthodontic band. To provide a pre-endodontic core restoration with an orthodontic band:

- Remove all the existing restorations and caries;
- Select a well-fitting orthodontic band;
- Place a cotton pledget directly over canal entrances to prevent cement blockage;
- Burnish the gingival margins of the band;
- Cement the chosen orthodontic band with a luting cement;
- Prepare an access cavity and remove the cotton pledget to uncover the root canal entrances.

Rubber dam

Rubber or dental dam isolation is mandatory for endodontic treatment. The main reasons for using rubber dam are to:

- Protect against the risk of inhalation of ingestion of endodontic instruments and irrigants;
- Eliminate microbial contamination, via saliva, of the exposed root canal system;
- Provide retraction of the soft tissues, e.g. buccal mucosa and tongue;
- Help improve comfort for the patient.

The essential rubber dam kit (Fig. 3.40a,b,c) comprises:

- Rubber dam
- Punch
- Clamps
- Clamp forceps
- Frame
- Dental floss or tape

Single tooth isolation

For the one-step technique (Fig. 3.41a,b,c,d,e):

- Punch a clean hole through the centre of the rubber dam;
- Floss through adjacent contact points;
- Select and try a winged clamp to ensure four-point contact around the base of the tooth (floss may be tied around the clamp, as a precaution, to aid retrieval of the clamp);
- Apply gentle pressure with a forefinger on the bow of the clamp to confirm stability;
- Remove the clamp;
- Place the clamp on top of the rubber dam and push the wings underneath the punched hole;
- Apply the rubber dam and clamp assembly with the forceps onto the tooth;
- Slip the rubber dam under the wings of the clamp with an instrument, e.g. a flat plastic;
- Place a paper napkin or tissue between the rubber dam and the patient's skin;
- Apply the frame;
- Apply a caulking/sealing agent, if necessary, to prevent leakage.

For the two-step technique (Fig. 3.42a,b,c):

- Punch a clean hole through the centre of the rubber dam;
- Floss through adjacent contact points;
- Select and try a winged or wingless clamp to ensure four-point contact around the base of the tooth (floss may be tied around the clamp, as a precaution, to aid retrieval of the clamp);
- Apply gentle pressure with a forefinger on the bow of the clamp to confirm stability;
- Stretch the rubber dam over the clamp and the tooth;

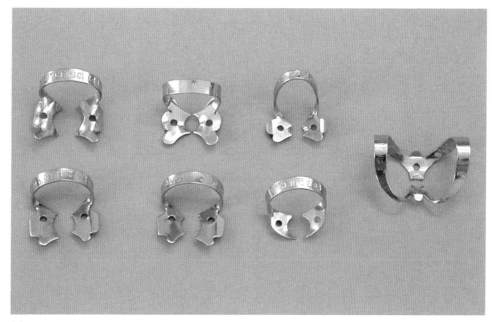

(a)

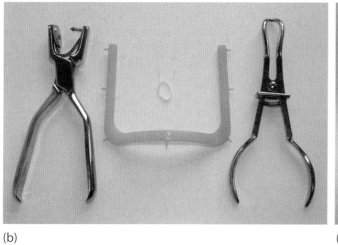

(b)

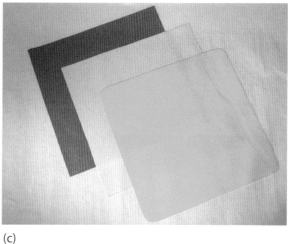

(c)

Figure 3.40 Rubber dam kit: (a) a selection of rubber dam clamps; (b) punch, forceps, frame, and dental floss; (c) selection of rubber dam sheets.

- Place a paper napkin or tissue between the rubber dam and the patient's skin;

- Apply the frame;

- Apply a caulking agent, if necessary, to prevent leakage.

Isolation of multiple teeth (split dam method)

When a tooth is broken down, there may not be sufficient sound tooth to retain a rubber dam clamp, or the clamps available may not be suitably shaped to give a firm, four-point contact around the tooth. In these situations, apart from building up a provisional core or temporary restoration as mentioned earlier, a neighbouring tooth may be used to retain the rubber dam clamp in what is known as the 'split dam' technique (Fig. 3.43a,b).

To isolate multiple teeth:

- Punch two clean holes through the rubber dam 5–7 mm apart, depending on the number and the size of the teeth to be isolated;

- Link the two punched holes by splitting the rubber in between with scissors;

- Floss through adjacent contact points;

- Select and try a winged or wingless clamps that give four-point contact around the gingival margins of the neighbouring tooth (floss may be tied around the clamp, as a precaution, to aid retrieval of the clamp);

- Apply gentle pressure with a forefinger on the bow of the clamp to confirm stability;

- Stretch the rubber dam over the clamp and the teeth;

- Place a paper napkin under rubber dam;

- Apply the frame.

Alternatively, once the rubber dam is in place, it may be secured by wedging the proximal contact points with tiny strips of rubber dam, rubber or silicone cords, or wooden wedges. If there are any signs of saliva leakage once the rubber dam is in place, then a caulking agent may be used.

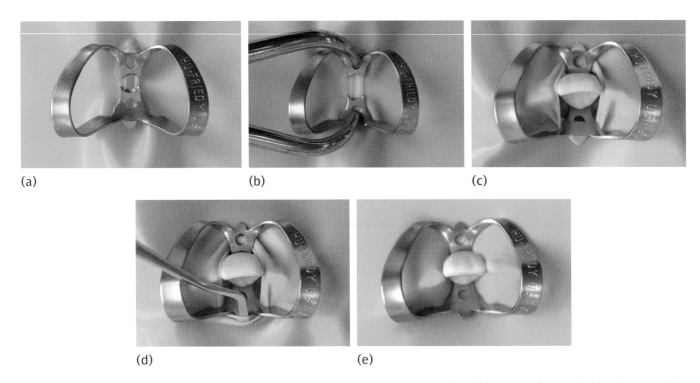

(a)　　　　　　　　　(b)　　　　　　　　　(c)

(d)　　　　　　　　　(e)

Figure 3.41 One-step rubber dam technique: (a) secure the clamp to the rubber dam using the wings; (b) open the clamp and rubber dam assembly using forceps; (c) rubber dam and clamp in place; (d) flick the rubber dam off the clamp wings using a flat plastic instrument; (e) rubber dam secured in position.

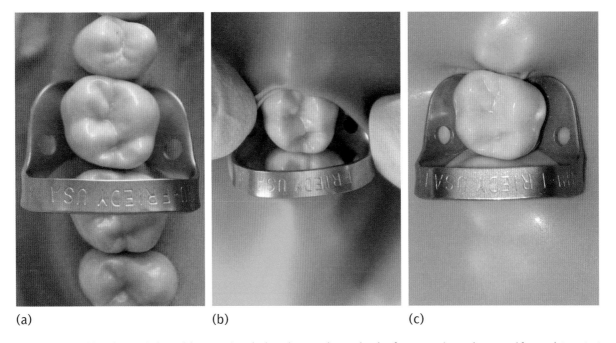

(a)　　　　　　　　　(b)　　　　　　　　　(c)

Figure 3.42 Two-step rubber dam technique: (a) secure the wingless clamp to the tooth using forceps and ensuring a good four-point contact; (b) stretch the rubber dam over the clamp; (c) rubber dam secured in position.

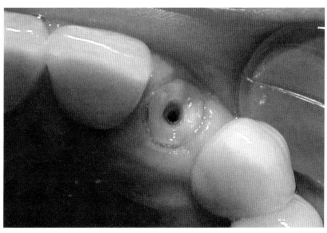

(a)

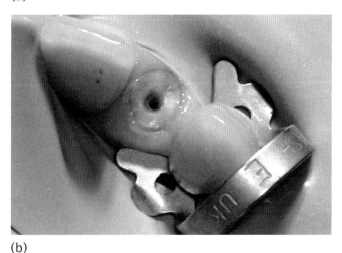

(b)

Figure 3.43 Clinical example of the split dam technique: (a) before placement and (b) the dam in place.

Summary points

- An accurate diagnosis is the key to successful treatment. The diagnostic process involves history taking, examination, and special investigations. Endodontic diagnosis involves identifying the status of pulpal and periapical tissues.

- History taking should involve open-ended, non-leading questions in order to obtain a full and accurate account of the patient's complaint; give an insight into the patient's motivation for, and expectation of, treatment; and identify any conditions which may dictate the need to modify treatment.

- The examination comprises extraoral and intraoral assessment. It should be thorough and systematic in order to identify any non-endodontic and endodontic disease.

- Special investigations may involve sensibility testing or radiographs. The former may include electric, cold, and heat tests; the latter may include conventional radiographs and cone beam computed tomography (CBCT).

- Once a diagnosis has been reached, a treatment plan can be formulated. This is a list of timetabled procedures individually tailored for the patient. It may be necessary to modify the treatment plan as treatment progresses.

- Common errors in endodontic diagnosis include misinterpretation of symptoms and signs which may appear to be endodontic in origin. It is important to rule of non-endodontic and even non-odontogenic causes.

- If a diagnosis cannot be reached, treatment should be delayed and consideration should be given to referring the patient to a specialist.

 Suggested further reading

Barnes JJ and Patel S (2011) Contemporary endodontics—part 1. *British Dental Journal* **211**, 463–8.

Bhuva B, Chong BS and Patel S (2008) Rubber dam in clinical practice. *Endodontic Practice Today* **2**, 131–41.

Chong BS (2010) *Harty's endodontics in clinical practice*, 6th edn. London: Churchill Livingstone.

European Society of Endodontology (2006) Quality guidelines for endodontic treatment: consensus report of the European Society of Endodontology. *International Endodontic Journal* **39**, 921–30.

Patel S and Horner K (2009) The use of cone beam computed tomography in endodontics. *International Endodontic Journal* **42**, 755–6.

Pitt Ford TR and Patel S (2004) Technical equipment for assessment of dental pulp status. *Endodontic Topics* **7**, 2–13.

Online Resource Centre

 To help you to develop and apply your knowledge and skills further, we have provided interactive learning resources online at http://www.oxfordtextbooks.co.uk/orc/patel/

4

Preserving pulp vitality

Avijit Banerjee

Chapter contents

Introduction

This chapter will introduce the underlying theory of preserving pulp vitality before exploring how this transfers to clinical practice. It is important that you read the whole chapter to understand how the theory and practice of preserving pulp vitality are related.

Why is vital pulp preservation important?

Endodontics involves preserving the vitality of the pulp, it is not just limited to pulp extirpation and root canal treatment. The preservation of pulp vitality underpins the successful practice of endodontics. The benefits of preserving pulp vitality are described in Chapter 2, and also summarized in Table 4.1. Root canal treatment is the last resort when the pulp tissue has become irreversibly inflamed and it is no longer healthy. However, there are steps a dentist can take to try to combat the caries process and prevent the need for this terminal treatment option.

Minimally invasive dentistry

Minimally invasive (MI) dentistry is an accepted operative caries treatment philosophy based upon the biological approach to caries excavation as opposed to a purely mechanistic, surgical approach taught for many years when dental amalgam was the material of choice for the majority of restorations. The understanding of the histopathology of the carious process has improved (Table 4.2). In addition, the successful development of adhesive materials with the ability to form a clinically acceptable *sealed* restoration means that some residual caries-affected dentine may be retained within the depths of the cavity during operative caries excavation procedures. It is essential that a peripheral border of sound enamel and/or sound or caries-affected dentine can be achieved. This, coupled with suitable operative parameters including adequate instrument access and moisture control measures, will result in the sealed-in residual caries-affected dentine arresting as the dentine–pulp complex defends against the disease process and is able to repair/remineralize the tooth structure. The methods by which the pulp can do this are outlined in Chapter 2.

When the carious process is within close proximity to the pulp (the shadow of the pulp can be seen through the thin dentine cavity floor) or may have breached the pulp (an exposure), clinical operative procedures can be considered in an attempt to protect the remaining pulp tissue from any further histological damage and permit healing, thus preserving the vitality of the pulpal tissues. However, for these measures to be successful certain important criteria must be met:

- The pulp must not have pre-existing symptoms of irreversible pulpitis;
- The pulp must exhibit positive responses to sensibility testing (see Chapter 3);
- Radiographic examination must reveal no signs of periapical periodontitis (e.g. widening of the periodontal ligament or periapical radiolucency).

Achieving a favourable outcome following these operative measures to protect the pulp are dependent upon:

- Removal of noxious stimuli;
- Stimulation of specific dentinogenic responses:
- Deposition of translucent (sclerotic) dentine at the advancing front of the lesion;

Table 4.1 Benefits of preserving the pulp

- To allow root development to continue in immature teeth (primary dentine formation)
- To maintain life-long tooth development (secondary dentine formation)
- To maintain the desirable physical properties of dentine (elasticity) by supplying nutrition to the organic components of dentine
- To maintain sensory function—nociception
- To maintain a defensive/protective role against caries, trauma, tooth surface loss

---

Table 4.2 Summary of the histological features of the zones of carious dentine.*

Caries-infected dentine (subjacent to enamel–dentine junction):
- Highly infected, necrotic bacterial biomass
- Soft, wet consistency due to gross demineralization
- Denatured collagen
- Loss of tubular structure
- Poor quality substrate to bond/seal/support the final restoration

Caries-affected dentine (deeper, towards the pulp):
- Bacterial load less than in infected dentine
- Less demineralization than infected dentine—scratchy and slightly sticky consistency to a sharp dental explorer
- Collagen partially damaged due to proteolysis
- Tubular structure more evident
- Has the potential to seal and support an adhesive restoration (especially if bordered with sound enamel)

* Note that these zones are separated for description only and that they blend in continuity from one to another without distinct boundaries.

- Deposition of reactionary or reparative tertiary dentine at the pulp–dentine interface;
- Immunoglobulins in the dentinal fluid;

- Prevention of future microleakage using sealed adhesive restoration which is maintained by the patient.

What procedures are available to preserve pulp vitality? (Table 4.3)

'Biological' caries excavation

Minimally invasive operative caries management dictates the complete removal of the soft, wet, necrotic caries-infected dentine (Table 4.2). Caries-infected dentine has a high bacterial load and is not a suitable substrate for achieving a seal or for physically supporting a restoration under load. Removal of caries-infected dentine can be accomplished using hand excavators, burs, and/or chemomechanical gel systems, e.g. Carisolv (Orasolv, Göteborg, Sweden). The colour of the dentine (usually dark brown, Fig 4.1) is not an indicator of the amount of tissue to be excavated, but instead, its tactile quality should be assessed. Caries-infected dentine is soft and sticky whereas the deeper caries-affected dentine has a scratchy-tacky texture to a sharp dental explorer. Peripheral excavation of the cavity should be carried out first in order to:

- Delineate the extent of the lesion in the tooth and to allow the clinical assessment of the remaining viable tooth structure (thus ascertaining the restorability of the tooth);
- To estimate the histological depth of the lesion (i.e. to assess the depth of infected, affected, and sound dentine using the sharp dental explorer without risking damage to the underlying pulp);
- To reveal a suitable dental substrate on which to achieve a peripheral adhesive seal.

Once this has been completed the caries overlying the pulp can be carefully excavated, again leaving caries-affected dentine only when the above listed criteria regarding the pathological signs/symptoms have been fulfilled. Finally, assuming suitable conditions exist for instrument access and moisture control, a sealed adhesive restoration can be placed and reviewed for any symptoms within 4–6 weeks. Evidence exists that if there are no signs or symptoms during this time period, it can be assumed that the dentine–pulp complex is winning its battle against the carious process, the lesion has arrested, and the remineralization process has begun. No radiographic changes will be evident at this stage.

The MI procedure known commonly as *stepwise excavation* (where the caries-infected dentine is removed superficially and a therapeutic lining plus provisional restoration are placed and then removed approximately 4–6 months later, further arrested dentine caries excavated and the definitive restoration placed) has now become superfluous. Clinical research evidence has shown that if the original restoration has sealed the residual caries successfully (no clinical signs/symptoms persist), there is no benefit gained by re-entering the cavity for further cavity preparation in a second visit. If glass ionomer cement (GIC) has been used for the initial sealed restoration, its occlusal surface may be veneered with resin composite six months or longer after placement.

Cavity linings and pulp protection

The concept of a separate therapeutic cavity lining to protect the pulp originated because dental amalgam, the restorative material of choice for many years, does not seal or interact chemically with the remaining cavity walls. Setting calcium hydroxide and zinc oxide-eugenol based cements have been used for many years as separate cavity liners but it is clear that neither of these types of materials fulfil many of the ideal properties required in contemporary operative dentistry. The ideal properties of a dental material used to protect the pulp are listed in Table 4.4. Modern adhesive restorative materials along with

Table 4.3 Summary of procedures to preserve pulp vitality

Procedure	Pulp exposed	Amount of pulp removed	Material used to protect the pulp
Biological caries excavation	No	None	Adhesive restoration (glass ionomer cement (GIC) or resin composite)
			If amalgam is definitive restoration, then use thin layer of GIC, or calcium silicate cement
Indirect pulp protection	No, but nearing an exposure	None	Adhesive restoration (GIC or resin composite)
			If amalgam is definitive restoration, then use thin layer of GIC
Direct pulp protection	Yes	None	Calcium silicate cement followed by an adhesive restoration
Partial coronal pulpotomy	Yes	Pulp removed until haemostasis achieved	Calcium silicate cement followed by an adhesive restoration
Coronal pulpotomy	Yes	All of coronal pulp	Calcium silicate cement followed by an adhesive restoration

the procedural steps used to achieve their adherent seal, often negate the need for a separate therapeutic lining material as they intrinsically exhibit many of the ideal properties listed in Table 4.4. This assumes that the adhesive materials are handled carefully and placed with the appropriate clinical technique. Therefore, the term 'cavity lining' should now be considered historical and the term 'pulp protection' used appropriately.

Indirect pulp protection (capping)

Indirect pulp protection is a procedure when residual caries-affected dentine is retained in close proximity to the pulp *without* an actual breach (exposure). The cavity is restored permanently with an

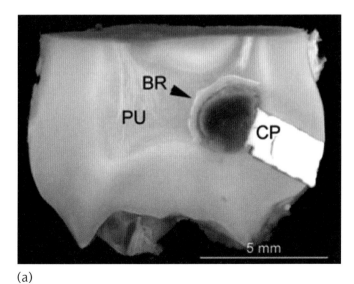

Figure 4.1 Caries affecting a maxillary first molar tooth. Note the dentine is dark brown. Caries-infected dentine will feel soft and sticky when explored.

Table 4.4 Ideal properties of a dental material used to protect the pulp
Protect the closely underlying pulp from: • Bacterial invasion (bacteriocidal) • Thermal/electrical stimuli (only relevant for overlying amalgam/metal-based restorations)
Stimulate the closely underlying pulp to produce: • Tertiary (reparative) dentine • Tertiary (regenerative) dentine to form a dentine bridge over an exposure • Anti-inflammatory cells chemical mediators
Prevent further long-term pulpal assault by: • Creating an adherent seal over the pulp so preventing microleakage • Reinforcing the remaining dentine by physico-chemical infiltration • Being present and active indefinitely to provide a physical support and barrier between the overlying restoration and the pulp • Being simple to place in the cavity, biocompatible with a long shelf life

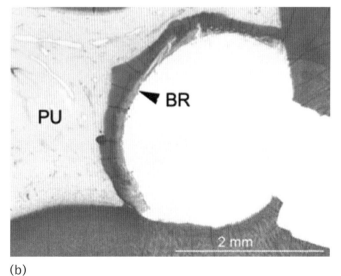

(a)   (b)

Figure 4.2 (a) Mesial half of a maxillary third molar showing the remnants of the restorative and direct Mineral Trioxide Aggregate pulp capping material (CP) and a distinct hard tissue bridge (BR) across the exposed pulp (PU). (b) Histological section of the dentine bridge (BR) formed across the exposed pulp (PU).

Adapted from Nair PNR, Duncan HF, Pitt Ford TR and Luder HU (2008) Histological, ultrastructural and quantitative investigations on the response of healthy human pulps to experimental capping with Mineral Trioxide Aggregate: a randomized controlled trial. *International Endodontic Journal* **41**, 128–50. Printed with permission from Wiley-Blackwell.

adhesive, sealed restoration, e.g. GIC and/or resin composite. If non-adherent amalgam is used as the definitive restoration, a thin layer of GIC can be placed as the 'indirect pulp capping' material of choice over the cavity floor closest to the pulp. The pulp status can be assessed at review appointments via the signs, symptoms, and sensibility testing. If an irreversible pulpitis develops after the tooth has been restored then root canal treatment will be indicated. The patient must be advised of this before commencing treatment. The advantage of indirect pulp protection is that it gives the dentine–pulp complex a chance to recover from the carious process, heal, and remineralize the remaining dentine whilst preserving the medium- to long-term vitality of the pulp and retain as much tooth structure as possible.

Direct pulp protection (capping)

Direct pulp protection involves managing the exposed surface of the pulp using a suitable material (direct pulp capping material) to try to stimulate dentine bridge formation to close over the exposure so repairing the breach (Fig. 4.2). Causes of pulp exposure include:

* Carious process (leading to an infected pulp);
* Dental trauma (depending on the injury sustained, pulp may or may not be infected);
* Iatrogenic (caused inadvertently by the clinician during cavity preparation—pulp often not infected).

The factors to be considered when deciding whether direct pulp protection would have a good prognosis include:

* The level of bacterial infection the pulp has sustained;
* The length of time the pulp has been affected;
* The histological status of the pulp (extrapolated from sensibility testing and dependent on the above two bullet points);
* The size of the breach (if greater than 2–3 mm, the prognosis is likely to deteriorate in a carious exposure);
* Achievable haemostasis (persistent haemorrhage is an indicator of an irreversibly damaged pulp).

There are several direct pulp capping materials available. Historically, setting calcium hydroxide cements have been the material of choice for direct pulp capping. This has now been superseded by calcium silicate cements, e.g. ProRoot MTA (Dentsply Tulsa Dental, Tulsa, OK, USA) (Fig. 4.3a), MTA-Angelus (Angelus, Londrina-PR, Brazil) or Biodentine (Septodont, Saint-Maur-des Fosses, France) (Fig. 4.3b). In the past it was thought that pulp capping materials mildly irritated and inflamed the exposed pulp surface so stimulating the differentiation of mesenchymal cells into odontoblasts resulting in the rapid production of reparative tertiary dentine. However, there is now evidence that indicates that bioactive molecules, including transforming growth factors (TGFs) and bone morphogenic proteins (BMPs), released from the dentine organic matrix by the action of the pulp capping materials, are responsible for the differentiation and upregulation of the odontoblasts.

Pulpotomy

This more invasive surgical procedure, with similar aims to direct pulp protection, involves removal of the inflamed coronal portion of the pulp tissue. Using a fine diamond bur in a rotary handpiece, the inflamed portion is amputated using the clinician's discretion until more healthy pulp tissue is exposed and haemostasis is readily achieved with moist cotton wool pledgets. The larger exposed surface is then dressed with a suitable direct pulp capping material and sealed with a well-adapted plastic restoration. There are different pulpotomy procedures, dependent upon the amount of pulp tissue removed:

* A *partial coronal (Cvek) pulpotomy* is removal of part of the coronal pulp;
* A *coronal pulpotomy* is removal of all of the coronal pulp.

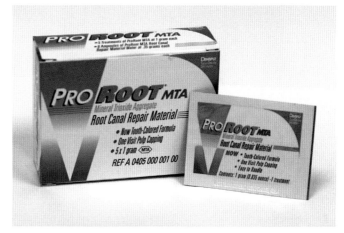

(a)

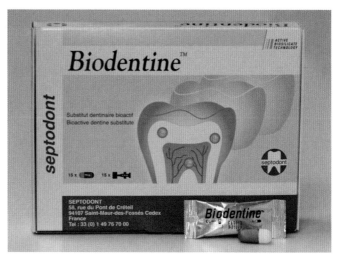

(b)

Figure 4.3 Calcium silicate cements: (a) ProRoot Mineral Trioxide Aggregate (MTA) (Dentsply Tulsa Dental, Tulsa, OK, USA); (b) Biodentine (Septodont, Saint-Maur-des Fosses, France).

Foundations of clinical practice

The remainder of this chapter will cover the practical aspects to carrying out vital pulp therapies. It will also discuss how to monitor the outcome of vital pulp therapies.

How do you carry out biological caries excavation?

The practical steps required to carry out biological caries excavation (Fig. 4.4) include:

- Check the occlusion preoperatively;
- Obtain a suitable shade match for the final tooth-coloured restoration;
- Administer local anaesthetic;
- Obtain suitable moisture control with rubber dam isolation;
- Gain access to the carious dentine through the enamel;
- Commence caries excavation at the enamel–dentine junction (EDJ) using rose-head burs in a slow speed handpiece or hand excavators. Carious, demineralized, unsupported enamel should be removed along with the soft, wet, and sticky caries-infected dentine. Ideally, sound dentine should be exposed at the periphery of the lesion along with sound enamel borders where possible, but there are instances when, if significant amounts of sound enamel is present, some caries-affected dentine might be retained even at the periphery (e.g. in occlusal cavities);
- Move towards the caries overlying the pulp and carefully excavate this with hand excavators. Chemomechanical gels may be useful in this situation to remove more selectively the infected, rather than affected, dentine;
- Gently wash and dry the final cavity;

- If amalgam is the restorative material of choice, then place a thin layer of GIC protection over the cavity floor closest to the pulp;
- Otherwise, restore the cavity with adhesive restorative materials (*GIC*—condition the cavity walls with 10 per cent polyacrylic acid for 15 seconds, wash, dry, place GIC, compact, shape, and finish once set; *resin composite*—apply dentine bonding agent following appropriate procedures for each type, layer photo-cured increments, finish).

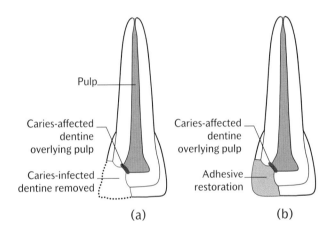

Figure 4.4 Biological caries excavation: (a) caries-affected dentine overlying the pulp is not excavated. (b) An adhesive restoration is placed over the caries-affected dentine without the need for an indirect pulp cap.

How do you carry out direct pulp protection (capping)?

The practical steps required to carry out direct pulp protection (Figs. 4.5 and 4.6) include:

- Check the occlusion preoperatively;
- Obtain a suitable shade match for the final tooth-coloured restoration;
- Administer local anaesthesia;
- Obtain moisture control with rubber dam isolation;
- If required, commence biological caries excavation as described above (this step is not necessary in the case of dental trauma). Clear all caries-infected and caries-affected dentine over the pulp, whilst trying to keep the size of the carious pulpal exposure as small as possible;
- Rinse the exposed pulp with 0.5 per cent sodium hypochlorite solution and then rinse with sterile, isotonic saline;

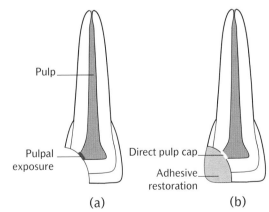

Figure 4.5 Direct pulp protection: (a) pulpal exposure and (b) direct pulp cap is placed over pulpal exposure. The tooth is restored with an adhesive restoration.

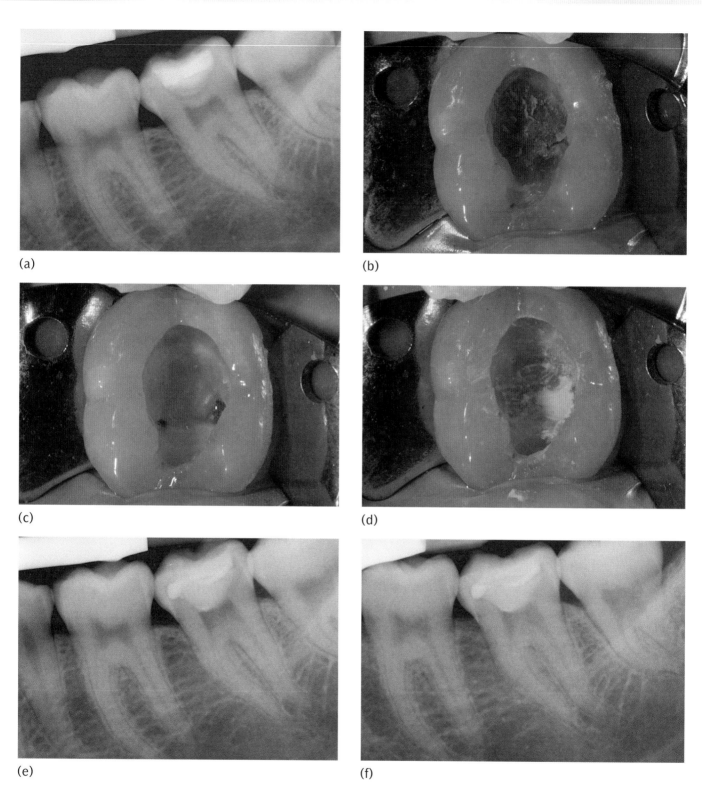

Figure 4.6 Direct pulp protection: (a) periapical radiograph of mandibular molar showing extent of carious lesion; (b) access is gained to caries-infected dentine; (c) pulpal exposure following caries excavation; (d) direct pulp cap using calcium silicate cement; (e) review periapical radiograph at 12 months; (f) review periapical radiograph at 36 months showing healthy periapical tissues.

- Pulp haemorrhage should stop after 2–3 minutes. It may be necessary to blot the pulp gently with a moist sterile cotton wool pledget to achieve haemostasis. Remove the blood clot;
- Place a direct pulp capping material over the pulpal exposure;
- If using Mineral Trioxide Aggregate (MTA) as the direct pulp cap, place a thin layer of GIC over the MTA, and restore the cavity definitively with a sealed adhesive restoration;

- If using Biodentine as the direct pulp cap, provisionally restore the entire cavity with Biodentine before veneering its occlusal surface definitively within six months with resin composite.

Persistent or extremes of bleeding (too much or too little) are usually a sign that the pulp damage is irreversible. In these cases a pulpotomy or pulpectomy procedure will be required. The prognosis of this procedure is affected adversely if the blood clot is not removed prior to application of the direct pulp capping material.

How do you carry out a pulpotomy?

The practical steps required to carry out a pulpotomy (Figs. 4.7 and 4.8) include:

- Check the occlusion preoperatively;
- Obtain a suitable shade match for the final tooth-coloured restoration;
- Administer local anaesthesia;
- Obtain moisture control with rubber dam isolation;
- If required, commence biological caries excavation as described above. Clear all the caries-infected and caries-affected dentine over the pulp;
- Rinse the exposed pulp with 0.5 per cent sodium hypochlorite solution and then rinse with sterile, isotonic saline;
- Remove the pulp in 1–2 mm increments using a diamond bur in a high-speed rotary handpiece with copious sterile water coolant until

excessive bleeding stops. Blood is removed with gentle irrigation with sterile saline and haemostasis achieved by blotting the pulp surface with moist sterile cotton wool pledgets;

- Place a suitable direct pulp capping material;
- If using MTA as the direct pulp cap, place a thin layer of GIC over the MTA, and restore the cavity definitively with a sealed adhesive restoration;
- If using Biodentine as the direct pulp cap, provisionally restore the entire cavity with Biodentine before veneering its occlusal surface definitively within six months with resin composite.

To prevent tearing and additional trauma to the already distressed pulp tissues, manual excavation or the use of steel burs in a slow-speed handpiece are contraindicated. For the same reason, dry cotton wool pledgets must never be used.

How do you monitor the outcome of vital pulp therapies?

It is important to review the vital pulp therapy within 6–12 months of treatment, and then annually for a further three years. The review should include patient's symptoms (if any), assessment of the pulpal and periapical status of the tooth, and the coronal seal of the overlying restoration. If a provisional restoration has been placed, this must be replaced with a definitive adhesive restoration as soon as possible to minimize the chances of marginal microleakage. Adhesive systems must be used carefully, always appreciating the vital interplay between the tooth substrate, the chemistry of the material, and the clinical handling procedures of both. Marginal integrity can be examined carefully using dental explorers ensuring no deficiencies develop and that the patient's oral hygiene procedures are adequate at removing the plaque biofilm from the restoration-tooth surface.

Criteria for a favourable outcome following pulp therapy

Clinical examination

- The patient should not suffer ongoing symptoms of pulpitis or periapical periodontitis;

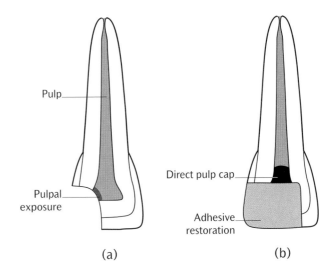

Figure 4.7 Pulpotomy: (a) traumatic pulpal exposure; (b) direct pulp cap is placed after removal of 2–3 mm of coronal pulp tissue. The tooth is restored with an adhesive restoration.

Adapted from Patel S and Duncan H (2011) *Pitt Ford's Problem-Based Learning in Endodontology.* Printed with permission from Wiley-Blackwell.

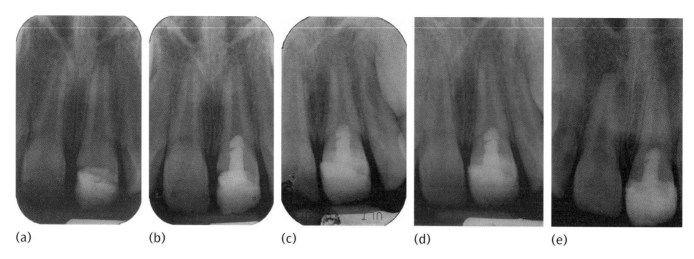

(a) (b) (c) (d) (e)

Figure 4.8 Pulpotomy of a previously traumatized maxillary incisor tooth: (a) preoperative radiograph; (b) immediately post-treatment; (c) 6 months; (d) 12 months; (e) 24 months.
Adapted from Patel S and Duncan H (2011) *Pitt Ford's Problem-Based Learning in Endodontology.* Printed with permission from Wiley-Blackwell.

- Within a few weeks, a positive response to sensibility testing should be elicited and the tooth and surrounding tissues should appear healthy, i.e. there should be no tenderness to percussion, if originally present.

Radiographic examination

- Immature teeth should show signs of further root development (compare to adjacent and contralateral teeth);

- The presence of a dentine bridge between the pulp and capping material (the absence of a bridge does not necessarily indicate an unfavourable outcome);

- Healthy periapical tissues (intact lamina dura and periodontal ligament).

Criteria for an unfavourable outcome following pulp therapy

Clinical examination

- No improvement, or worsening symptoms;

- Coronal discolouration and/or a negative response to sensibility testing;

- Further periapical involvement may be indicated by tenderness to palpation on the alveolar mucosa overlying the root apex, tenderness to percussion, presence of a sinus, or tooth mobility (periodontal alveolar bone levels should have been assessed preoperatively).

Radiographic examination

- Further widening of the periodontal ligament space;

- A developing periapical radiolucency.

Prognosis

Ultimately, the critical factors to be considered for a favourable prognosis of all vital pulp therapies include:

- **Using an aseptic technique**—using rubber dam isolation and sterile solutions to ensure the exposed pulp is not contaminated with microbes;

- **Control of pulp haemorrhage**—once haemostasis is achieved the blood clot must be removed carefully to permit the biochemical interaction between the pulp capping material and the vital pulp tissue;

- **Achieving a coronal seal**—this is imperative to prevent marginal microleakage.

Summary

The preservation of pulp vitality is dependent upon numerous factors outlined above. If dental disease (caries) is prevented or controlled, the dentine–pulp complex will not be significantly affected. However, it is also important to note that most invasive operative dentistry procedures (including cavity or crown preparation) can render the dentine–pulp complex at risk of irreversible damage from bacterial microleakage along freshly exposed dentine tubules and/or heat conduction from the operative procedure. It is therefore necessary for the clinician to appreciate the histology and materials being used to reduce the overall risk to the pulp.

Regular insults to the pulp reduce its recuperative powers and may lead to irreversible damage. Therefore, full consideration should be given to the removal of causative factors, whilst bearing in mind the possible consequences of the restorative procedures that may lead to future complications as a result of microleakage and the reduced remaining dentine thickness overlying the pulp. After pulp therapy is complete, a coronal seal must be achieved with an adhesive restoration, so preventing subsequent infection which could go undetected until the pulp status is irreversibly compromised.

Failure to achieve haemostasis is a clinical sign that the pulp may be irreversibly inflamed and/or infected, as indeed is very little or no haemorrhage. In these cases complete extirpation of the pulp (pulpectomy) will be necessary.

It is always wise to monitor the outcome of pulp preservation procedures on a periodic basis. In addition to checking signs/symptoms, sensibility testing should be carried out and an annual radiographic periapical examination may show signs of dentine bridge formation as well as no periapical changes.

In immature teeth, the vitality of the pulp should be preserved, when possible, to allow for further root development. In fully mature teeth, root canal treatment is usually the treatment of choice if there is any doubt of the vitality of the pulp and/or there has been a carious pulpal exposure. This is especially relevant when the tooth is to be restored with an extensive restoration (e.g. a multi-surface class 2 composite restoration or a cuspal coverage restoration). There is evidence to suggest that the incidence of loss of vitality is higher in these teeth when compared to teeth restored with less extensive restorations.

Summary points

- Clinicians should take a biological approach to caries removal and pulp protection.
- Clinicians should consider vital pulp therapies when possible, especially in vital immature teeth to allow for further root development.
- Vital pulp therapies are contraindicated in teeth with irreversible pulpitis or teeth with large carious pulpal exposures.
- Procedures available to preserve pulp vitality include: biological caries excavation, direct pulp protection and pulpotomy.
- Contemporary pulp protection materials include calcium silicate cements and adhesive restorative materials.

 Suggested further reading

Ainehchi M, Eslami B, Ghanbariha M and Saffar AS (2003) Mineral Trioxide Aggregate (MTA) and calcium hydroxide as pulp-capping agents in human teeth: a preliminary report. *International Endodontic Journal* **36**, 225-31.

Banerjee A and Watson TF (2011) *Pickard's Manual of Operative Dentistry*, 9th edn. Oxford, UK: Oxford University Press.

Bjørndal L, Reit C, Bruun G, Markvart M, Kjaeldgaard M, Näsman P, Thordrup M, Dige I, Nyvad B, Fransson H, Lager A, Ericson D, Petersson K, Olsson J, Santimano EM, Wennström A, Winkel P and Gluud C (2010) Treatment of deep carious lesions in adults: randomized clinical trials comparing stepwise vs. direct complete excavation, and direct vs. partial pulpotomy. *European Journal of Oral Sciences* **118**, 290-7.

Cox CF, Bergenholtz G, Fitzgerald M, Heys DR, Heys RJ, Avery JK andBaker JA (1982) Capping of the dental pulp mechanically exposed to the oral microflora—a 5 week observation of wound healing in the monkey. *Journal of Oral Pathology* **11**, 327–39.

Cox CF, Bergenholtz G, Heys DR, Syed SA, Fitzgerald M and Heys RJ (1985) Pulp capping of dental pulp mechanically exposed to oral microflora: a 1–2 year observation of wound healing in the monkey. *Journal of Oral Pathology* **14**, 156–68.

Nair PN, Duncan HF, Pitt Ford TR and Luder HU (2008) Histological, ultrastructural and quantitative investigations on the response of healthy human pulps to experimental capping with Mineral Trioxide Aggregate: a randomized controlled trial. *International Endodontic Journal* **41**, 128–50.

Smith AJ, Murray PE and Lumley PJ (2002) Preserving the Vital Pulp in Operative Dentistry: 1. A Biological Approach . *Dental Update* **29**, 64–9.

Swift EJ, Trope M and Ritter AV (2003) Vital pulp therapy for the mature tooth—can it work? *Endodontic Topics* **5**, 49–56.

Online Resource Centre

 To help you to develop and apply your knowledge and skills further, we have provided interactive learning resources online at http://www.oxfordtextbooks.co.uk/orc/patel/

5

Root canal preparation

Edward Brady and Conor Durack

Chapter contents

Introduction

This chapter will introduce the rationale for root canal preparation before exploring how this transfers to clinical practice. It is important that you read the whole chapter to understand how the theory and practice of root canal preparation are related.

What is root canal treatment and why do it?

Root canal treatment involves the removal of pulpal tissue and the disinfection of the root canal system. The disinfected root canal system is then sealed to prevent the re-entry and growth of microbes. The ultimate objective of treatment is to restore and maintain periapical health, enabling the tooth to be preserved as a healthy, functional unit within the dental arch.

The indications for root canal treatment are:

- Irreversible inflammation of the pulp;
- An infected necrotic pulp (usually with evidence of periapical periodontitis);
- Pulpal necrosis (e.g. after a traumatic injury to the tooth);
- Elective root canal treatment is sometimes indicated as part of a restorative treatment plan, usually in circumstances where the root canal space is required for the retention of a coronal restoration, e.g. a post-retained crown.

Root canal treatment is carried out in two stages:

- Root canal preparation;
- Root canal filling (see Chapter 6).

What are the aims of root canal preparation?

Root canal preparation involves simultaneous mechanical and chemical preparation of the root canal system (chemomechanical debridement). The aims of chemomechanical debridement are to:

- Remove microbes;
- Remove pulpal remnants and organic debris, which provide a substrate for microbes;
- Create an optimal shape to allow a well-compacted root canal filling to be placed into the root canal system.

What are the aims of mechanical preparation?

Mechanical preparation is achieved using a variety of instruments (both manual and machine driven) to clean and shape the root canal system. The ideal prepared root canal shape is a three-dimensional continuously tapering cone, which is narrowest apically and widest at the root canal entrance. The taper should ideally be centred along the original axis of the root canal and maintain the original contour (Fig. 5.1).

The aims of mechanical preparation are:

- The removal of pulpal debris and microbes;
- To provide a suitable shape for effective irrigation of the root canal system;
- To provide improved access for the placement of medicaments;
- To provide the optimal shape and resistance form for the root canal filling.

Contemporary instrumentation of the root canal is carried out using a 'crown-down' approach: the coronal portion of the root canal is initially instrumented and flared before progressing apically with instruments.

What are the aims of chemical preparation?

Successful root canal treatment is dependent upon the elimination (as far as possible) of infection from the root canal system. This is achieved by chemical preparation using:

- Antimicrobial irrigants;
- Interappointment medicaments.

The root canal system is irrigated with antimicrobial solutions during mechanical preparation. Frequent, copious irrigation is essential if successful cleaning and disinfection are to be achieved. Medicaments are used to dress the root canal system between visits to further reduce the levels of microbes in the root canal system.

The aims of chemical preparation are:

- To flush out remnants of pulp tissue and debris created during mechanical instrumentation;
- To dissolve residual pulpal tissue;

- To kill microbes and remove microbial biofilm;
- To clean the parts of the root canal system which are inaccessible (e.g. isthmi and lateral canals) to mechanical instrumentation;
- To facilitate instrumentation and prevent root canal blockages by acting as a lubricant;
- To remove the smear layer.

Effective chemical preparation is the most important aspect of root canal preparation. Although in recent years there have been great advances in equipment and techniques available for mechanical preparation, the importance of effective chemical preparation must not be overlooked.

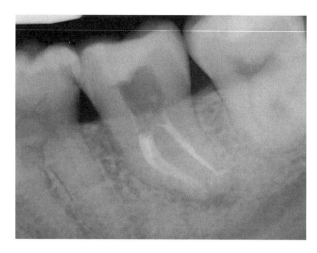

Figure 5.1 An endodontically treated mandibular molar tooth: note the uniform taper of the root canal fillings and how they follow the root outline.

What are the challenges encountered during root canal preparation?

The anatomy of the root canal system can be very complex (Fig. 5.2). Several factors may present a challenge to effective mechanical instrumentation:

- In addition to the main root canal(s), there are accessory canals, lateral canals, fins, anastomoses, isthmi, and apical deltas, all of which are inaccessible to mechanical instrumentation.

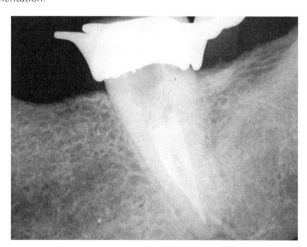

Figure 5.2 An endodontically treated mandibular molar tooth: note that the isthmus between the root canals has been filled.

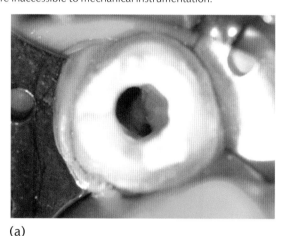

(a)

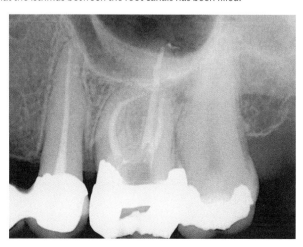

Figure 5.3 Severe root canal curvature.

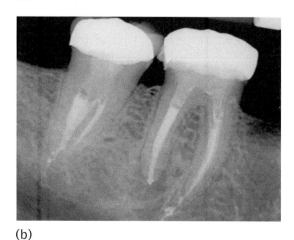

(b)

Figure 5.4 Mandibular second molar with a C-shaped root canal: (a) intraoperative clinical appearance and (b) postoperative radiographic appearance.

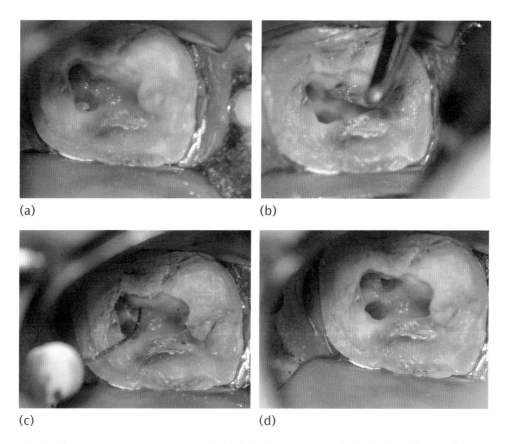

(a)　　　　　　　　(b)

(c)　　　　　　　　(d)

Figure 5.5 Second mesio-buccal root canal in a maxillary molar tooth: (a) clinical appearance prior to location, (b) ultrasonic tips utilized to locate entrance to root canal, (c) initial instrumentation of root canal, (d) clinical appearance after root canal preparation.

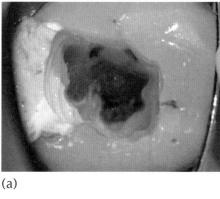

(a)

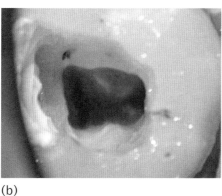

(b)

Figure 5.6 Pulp stones (a) before and (b) after removal.

- Root canals may have severe or double (S-shaped) curvatures (Fig. 5.3), which may not be readily detectable on radiographs. These present a challenge to instrumentation, as the some of instruments used for root canal preparation are straight and can be inflexible.

- The cross-section of root canals are frequently oval or ribbon shaped; some molar teeth have C-shaped root canals (Fig. 5.4a,b).

- Instruments are usually uniform in cross-section and are unable to fully contact all surfaces of the root canals.

- Teeth often have a greater number of root canals than anticipated. For example, the mesio-buccal roots of maxillary molars frequently have two root canals (Fig. 5.5a,b,c,d).

- Deposition of secondary and tertiary dentine may result in partially or completely calcified root canals. Pulp stones and dystrophic calcifications may also be encountered (Fig. 5.6).

- Patient factors such as restricted mouth opening may preclude endodontic treatment of posterior teeth. A strong gag reflex can complicate the placement of rubber dam and the taking of periapical radiographs.

- The position and angulation of the tooth may affect the feasibility of endodontic treatment

- Existing restorations may mask the true orientation of the tooth and lead to procedural errors when attempting to locate the root canals.

What are the stages in mechanical preparation?

Mechanical preparation can be divided into the following stages:

- Preparation of the tooth for root canal treatment;
- Access cavity preparation and location of root canal entrances;
- Creating straight-line access;
- Initial negotiation;
- Coronal flaring;
- Working length determination;
- Apical preparation.

Preparation of the tooth for root canal treatment

Before embarking on treatment, a thorough clinical and radiographic assessment needs to be made to determine the restorability of the tooth and to predict any difficulties which may be encountered during treatment. Caries and defective restorations must be removed. If there is any doubt regarding the restorability of the tooth, all restorations should be removed to allow a full assessment to be made. It is frequently necessary to place a provisional restoration or to provide support for undermined cusps prior to embarking on treatment. Time spent on this stage of the procedure will save much time and stress later on.

Access cavity preparation, location of root canals, and creating straight-line access

The first stage of root canal treatment is the preparation of an access cavity and the location of the root canal entrances. This stage is frequently the most difficult part of root canal treatment but if carried out proficiently, it will allow the subsequent preparation of the root canals to progress much more smoothly. It is important to be familiar with tooth morphology (Fig 5.7). Awareness of the usual position of the pulp chamber, the number of root canals, and the location of root canal entrances reduces unnecessary removal of tooth structure during access cavity preparation and reduces the possibility that any root canals will be missed.

Once the root canal entrances have been located, straight-line access to the root canals must be established. Straight-line access (Fig. 5.8) is important because:

- It reduces stress on instruments thus reducing the chance of instrument fracture;
- It reduces the chance of procedural errors (Fig. 5.9a,b,c,d,e);
- It simplifies treatment by providing a clear path of insertion for the instruments.

Initial negotiation and coronal flaring

Once the root canal has been located, the coronal half to two-thirds of the root canal is negotiated and instrumented to produce a tapered preparation, which is widest coronally (Fig. 5.10). At this stage, it is not necessary to instrument the apical portion of the root canal.

The advantages of coronal flaring prior to apical preparation are:

- Removal of coronal obstructions to enable unrestricted access to the apical portion of the root canal;
- Straightening of the coronal portion of the root canal;
- Better tactile feedback for instrumentation apically;
- Removal of the bulk of infected pulpal tissue and debris to prevent coronal microbes and debris from being introduced into the apical portion of the root canal;
- To provide a reservoir for irrigant coronally;
- To minimize the risk of creating apical blockages;
- Maintenance of working length during subsequent preparation.

Apical negotiation and working length determination

After coronal flaring has been completed, the apical portion of the root canal is negotiated and the working length is determined.

What is the working length?

The working length is the length of the root canal preparation, measured from a suitable coronal reference point (e.g. cusp tip or incisal edge), to the estimated position of the apical constriction. Straightening of the coronal portion of the root canal during coronal flaring often causes a slight reduction in the working length, so the working length determination should be carried out after coronal flaring.

How is the working length determined?

There are two main techniques for working length determination:

- Radiograph technique;
- Electronic apex locator (EAL) technique.

When using the radiographic technique, the working length is first estimated from a preoperative radiograph. This can be measured directly on the radiograph if film is being used, or if a digital radiographic system is employed, it may be measured using the radiograph viewing software. A file is placed into the root canal at this estimated length, and a parallel periapical radiograph is taken to determine the distance of the file tip from the radiographic apex.

The electronic apex locator (EAL) is attached to a file inserted into the root canal, which is gradually moved apically until the file reaches the apical foramen. This is indicated on the display and is referred to as the 'zero reading' (displayed as either 'APEX', 'red segment' or '0' depending on the EAL device). The technique for using an apex locator is described later in this chapter.

Both of the above methods for the determination of working length are reliable and may be used alone. Electronic apex locators are exceptionally useful for quick determination of the working length and are generally accurate, but a working length radiograph provides additional

Maxillary teeth	Root length	Number of canals	Features	Access cavity
				Buccal — Distal——+——Mesial — Palatal
1	23	1	• Access starting at cingulum and extend towards incisal edge	
2	22	1	• Triangular shape to encompass pulp horns • Lateral insisor-apical 3-4 mm has palatal curvature which should always be borne in mind when instrumenting	
3	26	1	• Canine-rounder access cavity then incisors-no need to flare access cavity as there is only 1 pulp horn	
4	21	1–5% 2–90% (B, P) 3–5% (MB, DB, P)	• Initial point of access should be centre of occlusal central groove • Widen access bucco-palatally to locate root canal entrance under respective cusp tips (P and B) • Second premolars if only one root canal then should be centred and oval in shape (bucco-palatally) to encompass pulp horns	
5	21	1–75% 2–25% (B, P)	• Second premolars root canal entrance more centred, if not centred look for second entrance under other cusp tip • Separate root canals join apically commonly	
6	22	P longer than MB and DB 3–40% (MB, DB, P) 4–60% (MB1, MB2, DB, P)	• Rhomboid access cavity outline • Distal apect of access cavity is on the mesial aspect of transverse ridge • Palatal root canal entrance is usually the largest and therefore easiest to locate • Disto-buccal and palatal root canal entrances usually rounder • Mesio-buccal root canal entrance usually more ovoid, reflecting ribbon shape of the mesio-buccal root • MB2 located between MB1 and palatal root canal • Troughing this area with fine burs or ultrasonic tips should eventually reveal an opening of a root canal entrance	
7	20	P longer than MB and DB 3–60% (MB, DB, P) 4–40% (MB1, MB2, DB, P)	• Lower incidence of MB2 in second molars • DB root canal closer to centre of tooth in second and third molars • Increased likelihood of fusion of root canals in second and third molars (1 buccal and 1 palatal)	

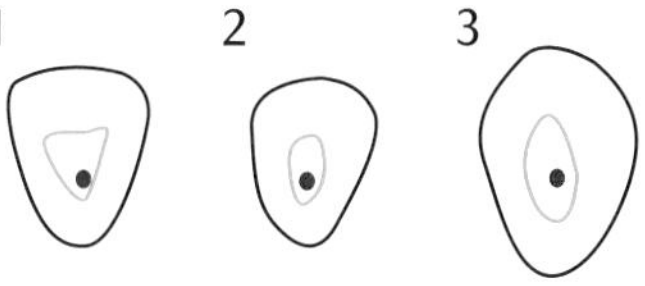

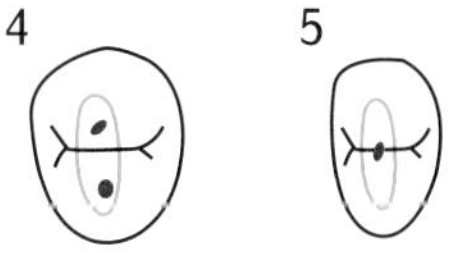

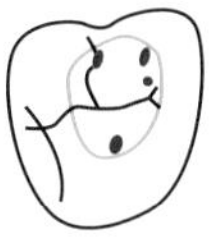

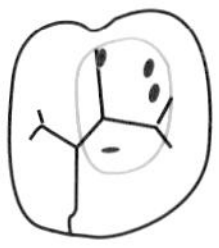

Mandibular teeth	Root length	Number of canals	Features	Access cavity
				Buccal — Distal——+——Mesial — Lingual
1	21	1–60% 2–40% (B, L)	• Starts at the base of the cingulum • Access cavity should be extented nearly to incisal edge to confirm the presence/absence of the second (lingual) root canal	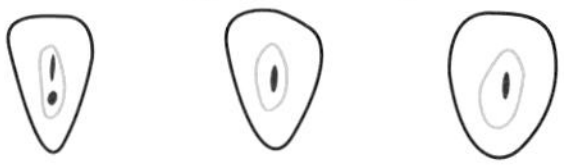
2	21			
3	24	1–90% 2–10% (B, L)	• Starts at the base of the cingulum	
4	22	1–75% 2–25% (B, L)	• Starts in central occlusal groove • Access is oval bucco-lingually in shape	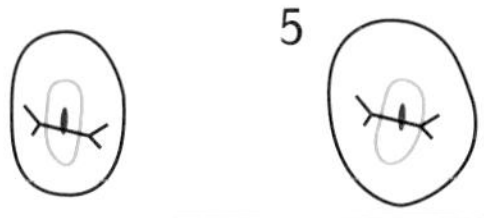
5	22	1–90% 2–10% (B, L)		
6	21	3–65% (ML, MB, D) 4–35% (ML, MB, DL, DB)	• Mesial root canal entrances are found below respective cusp tips • Larger distal root canal entrance is more centred • If distal root canal entrance is not centred then there is an increased likelihood of a second root canal • Increased incidence of fused root canals with second and third molars	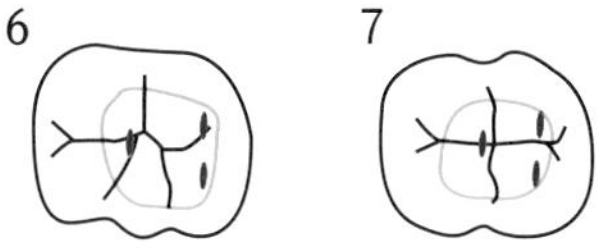
7	20	3–90% (MB, ML, D) 2–10% (M, D)		

B, buccal; P, palatal; MB, mesio-buccal; DB, disto-buccal; MB1, first mesio-buccal; MB2, second mesio-buccal; L, ligual; ML, mesio-ligual; D, distal; DL, distol-lingual.

Figure 5.7 Root canal features, average lengths, and access cavities in various teeth.

information, such as root canal curvature, that cannot be obtained using an EAL alone. For optimal accuracy, it is recommended that a combination of the two methods is utilized.

Other techniques have been advocated for working length determination. These include the use tactile feedback to feel for the apical

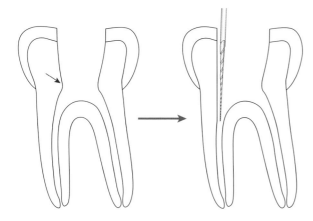

Figure 5.8 Refinement of access cavity to obtain straight-line access to mesial root canals of a mandibular molar. Overhanging dentine (red arrow) prevents straight-line access into the root canal.

constriction, and the insertion of a paper point into the root canal beyond the apex to pick up moisture/blood. The length of the dry section of the paper point gives some indication of the working length. Other techniques are not sufficiently reliable to be used exclusively, but may be useful when used in conjunction with other methods.

What is the terminus for the root canal preparation?

Preparation and subsequent root canal filling should end at the apical constriction (the narrowest part of the root canal). On average, this point lies approximately 0.5–1.0 mm short of the apical foramen (Fig. 5.11). Once the distance to the apical foramen is known (the zero reading given by an apex locator), 0.5–1.0 mm can be subtracted to give a working length that should terminate at, or very close to, the apical constriction. The apical foramen is not always located at the radiographic apex of the root and may in some instances be located up to 3 mm from the radiographic apex.

Apical preparation

After working length determination, apical preparation may be completed. The aim is to produce a tapered preparation, which tapers smoothly into the coronal preparation (Fig. 5.12). When preparing

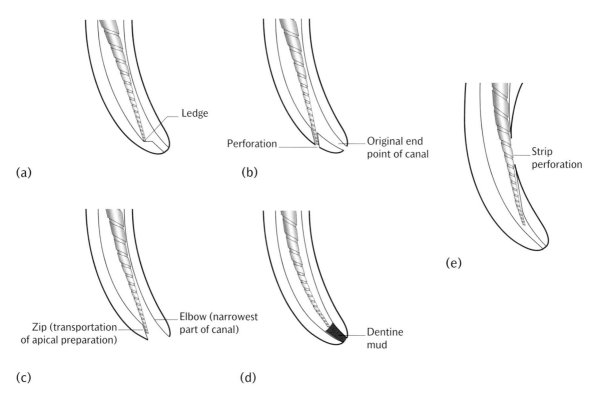

Figure 5.9 Root canal procedural errors: (a) ledge, (b) perforation, (c) zip and elbow formation, (d) apical blockage, (e) strip perforation.

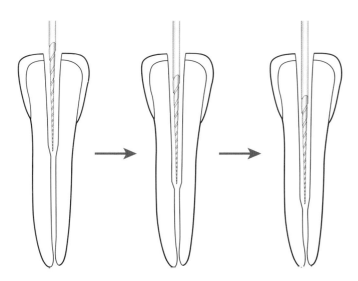

Figure 5.10 Coronal flaring.

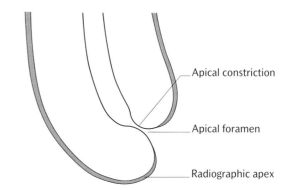

Figure 5.11 Relationship between the apical constriction, apical foramen, and radiographic apex of the root.

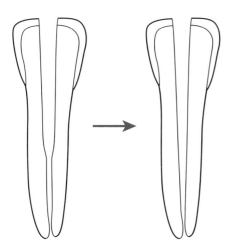

Figure 5.12 Diagram showing transition from coronally flared root canal to apically prepared root canal.

the root canal with stainless steel files, apical preparation involves two stages:

- Apical enlargement;
- Creation of apical taper.

Apical enlargement is necessary to allow adequate space for the penetration and exchange of irrigant and for the placement of medicaments. Creation of apical taper produces an optimal shape for effective irrigation and root canal filling. When using nickel-titanium (NiTi) files the apical size and taper are produced by the finishing file specific to the chosen system.

What should the size of the apical preparation be?

The size of the apical preparation is determined by the initial (pre-treatment) size of the root canal at the apex. Stainless steel files are inserted passively into the root canal to the working length to determine the apical diameter of the root canal. This process is known as 'gauging'. In situations where the root canal is initially very narrow, a decision has to be made regarding how large the apical preparation should be.

Controversy exists over the ideal size of the apical preparation, and recommendations vary from school to school. Generally, the accepted minimum size of apical preparation is ISO size 25, but frequently, larger sizes are advocated. Root canal curvature often dictates the maximum acceptable size, especially if stainless steel files are used. The proposed advantages of larger sized apical preparations are:

- Greater removal of infected dentine in the apical portion of the root canal;
- Improved irrigant exchange and access for medicaments in the apical portion of the root canal;
- Easier insertion of gutta-percha (GP) points to the working length, and creation of an apical 'stop'.

The potential disadvantages of larger sized apical preparations are the increased risk of procedural errors especially in severely curved root canals, and the extrusion of irrigant or root canal filling materials.

What is patency filing?

Patency filing refers to the passive placement of a small hand file, (ISO size 10 or smaller) 0.5–1.0 mm through the apical constriction during root canal preparation. The aim of patency filing is to prevent blockage of the apical portion of the root canal by debris created during instrumentation. A potential drawback of patency filing is that infected debris might be extruded into the periapical tissues, resulting in a postoperative flare-up.

What equipment and instruments are used for root canal preparation?

General equipment and instruments

Rubber dam

The use of rubber dam during root canal treatment is mandatory. Rubber dam protects the patient from accidental inhalation of instruments or irrigant, it prevents infection of the root canal from the oral cavity, retracts the soft tissues to provide a clear operating field, and greatly improves patient comfort. The use of rubber dam will ultimately allow root canal treatment to be carried out more effectively and predictably.

Magnification and illumination

Good visibility is essential when carrying out root canal treatment. The use of dental loupes equipped with a light (Fig. 5.13) or a dental

Electronic apex locators

Electronic apex locators (EALs) are used to determine the working length (Fig. 5.19). They work by setting up a local electric current between the patient's oral mucosa and the periodontal ligament at the end of the root canal. It is assumed that the electrical resistance of the periodontal ligament is the same as the oral mucosa. The apex locator has two terminals: a hook, which rests on the patient's lip, and a clip, which attaches to the file in the root canal. The EAL measures the resistance between the file in the root canal and the oral mucosa. When the file makes initial contact with the periodontal ligament outside the root canal, the display will give a zero reading, which is used to decide where the apical preparation will end. Apex locators are extremely useful and

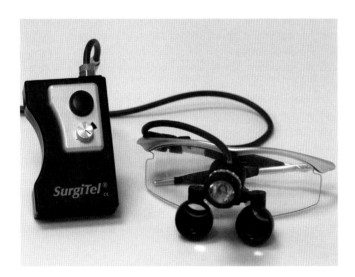

Figure 5.13 Dental loupes (SurgiTel, Ann Arbor, MI, USA).

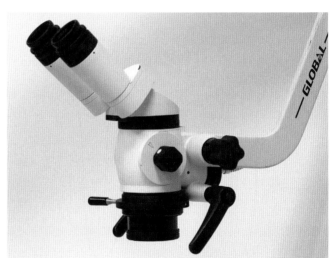

Figure 5.14 Dental operating microscope (Global Surgical, St Louis, MO, USA).

operating microscope (Fig. 5.14) greatly assists in the location of the entrances of root canals, and in the diagnosis of cracks and perforations.

Electric motor and speed reducing handpiece

Electric motors and speed reducing handpieces (Fig. 5.15) are used in conjunction with rotary or reciprocating NiTi files. Rotary electric motors are usually operated at between 150 and 500 rpm and allow the control of the torque to reduce the risk of file fracture. Speed reducing handpieces that operate on a standard slow-speed motor are also available, some of which offer limited torque control. However, they usually do not allow such precise control over speed and torque as an electric motor.

Ultrasonic units and tips

Piezo-electric ultrasonic units (Fig. 5.16) may be used in conjunction with dedicated endodontic tips (Fig. 5.17) for the removal of controlled amounts of dentine. They may also be used with an ultrasonic file attached (Fig. 5.18) to agitate irrigant in the root canal (passive ultrasonic irrigation).

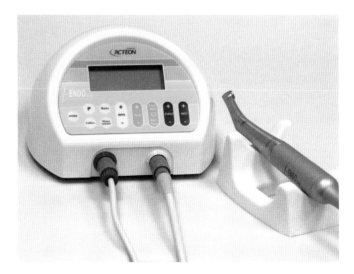

Figure 5.15 Endodontic motor: I-Endo dual (SATELEC ACTEON, Merignac, France).

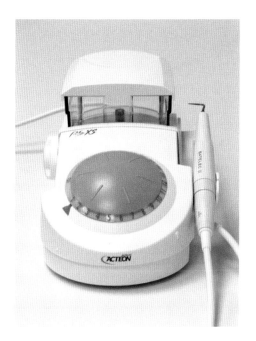

Figure 5.16 Ultrasonic device: P5 Newtron XS (SATELEC ACTEON, Merignac, France).

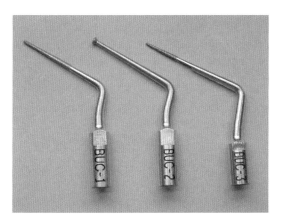

Figure 5.17 BUC ultrasonic tips (SybronEndo, Orange, CA, USA).

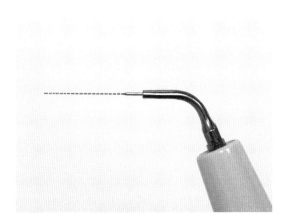

Figure 5.18 Ultrasonic file for passive ultrasonic irrigation.

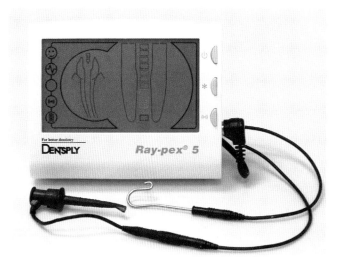

Figure 5.19 Electronic apex locator (EAL): Ray-pex 5 (DentsplyVDW, Munich, Germany).

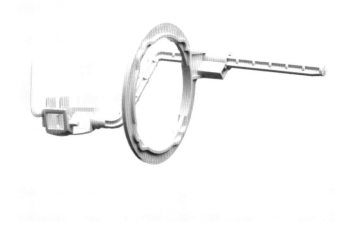

Figure 5.20 Endodontic film holder: EndoRay (Dentsply Rinn, Elgin, IL, USA).

are generally reliable but if any doubt exists as to the accuracy of the reading given, a supplementary technique should be used for working length determination.

Endodontic radiograph holders

Taking radiographs during endodontic treatment with rubber dam in place can be challenging. Specialized radiograph film or sensor holders are available to make the process of taking radiographs more reliable (Fig. 5.20). The holders include a beam aiming device and a basket to accommodate endodontic files and the rubber dam clamp.

Front surface mirror

Front surface mirrors have a reflective surface at the front of the glass, which means they do not produce a double image as standard mirrors do (Fig. 5.21a,b).

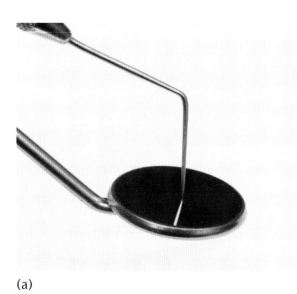

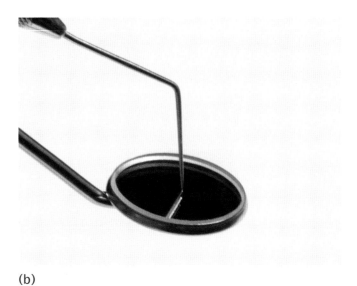

(a)   (b)

Figure 5.21 (a) Front surface mirror and (b) Standard dental mirror, note the double image.

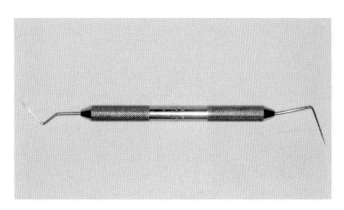

Figure 5.22 Endodontic explorer: DG16 (ASH Instruments, Dentsply, Addlestone, UK).

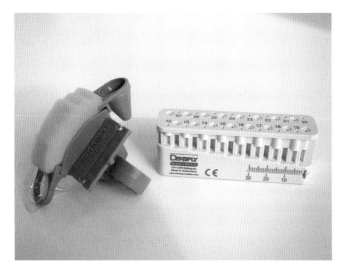

Figure 5.23 Selection of measuring devices (left to right): Endo Ring (SybronEndo, Orange, CA, USA), Endo Block (Dentsply-Maillefer, Ballaigues, Switzerland). The Endo Ring is a useful device because it has an incorporated sponge to hold files and clean debris from the flutes.

Endodontic explorer

The endodontic explorer is a double-ended probe with long, sharp tips (Fig. 5.22). This is useful for the location of root canal entrances.

Locking tweezers

Locking tweezers are ideal for gripping paper and GP points and for passing these between the dental nurse and clinician.

Long shank excavator

A long shank excavator is used to remove pulp stones and debris from the floor of the pulp chamber.

Measuring device

Various measuring devices are available for measurement of files, irrigating needles, and GP points (Fig, 5.23).

Burs for access cavity preparation

Tungsten carbide or diamond burs may be used for initial access cavity preparation. Tungsten carbide burs are more efficient when cutting through metallic restorations, but diamond burs should be used for cutting through ceramic, as they are less likely to cause fracture. Safe ended burs allow lateral extension of the access cavity outline after initial penetration without damaging the floor of the pulp chamber. Long shank burs may be used to remove tertiary dentine when attempting to locate root canal entrances (Fig. 5.24).

Instruments used for mechanical preparation

Gates Glidden drills

Gates Glidden drills are side cutting stainless steel instruments with non-cutting tips, which may be used to flare the coronal portion of the root canal (Fig. 5.25 and Table 5.1). They are manufactured in six sizes indicated by the number of bands on the shank of the instrument. Due to their inflexibility, they can only be used in the straight part of

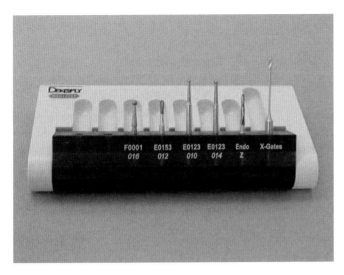

Figure 5.24 Cavity access set (Dentsply-Maillefer, Ballaigues, Switzerland).

Table 5.1 Gates Glidden drills and their corresponding ISO file sizes

Size	ISO size equivalent	Diameter (mm)
1	50	0.5
2	70	0.7
3	90	0.9
4	110	1.1
5	130	1.3
6	150	1.5

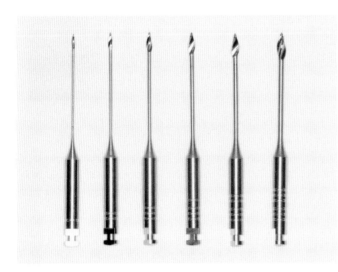

Figure 5.25 Selection of Gates Glidden drills.

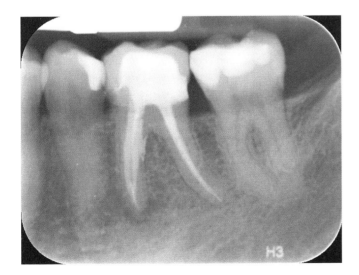

Figure 5.26 Strip perforation of mesial root.

the root canal. They have a long shank that is designed to fracture at the neck. This means that if they break they are usually easily retrievable, although this is not always the case. Gates Glidden drills have a very aggressive cutting action and if not used judiciously, are liable to remove excessive amounts of dentine, especially if sizes four and above are used. This can result in strip perforations, especially in narrow roots, such as the mesial roots of mandibular molars (Fig. 5.26).

Stainless steel files

Traditionally, endodontic files have been manufactured from stainless steel (Fig. 5.27). Stainless steel is flexible at smaller sizes (ISO size < 20), but at larger sizes, stiffness markedly increases. This can result in procedural errors (Fig. 5.9a,b,c,d,e). An advantage of stainless steel files is that at smaller sizes, they can be pre-curved to facilitate the negotiation of sharp curvatures (Fig. 5.28). Their rigidity is also invaluable in the initial negotiation of calcified root canals.

Stainless steel files used today (e.g. K-Flexofile, K-Flex, Hedström) are manufactured to a tip size and taper standardized by the International Organization for Standardization (ISO). The number associated with an ISO standard sized file refers to its tip diameter in one-hundredths of a millimetre, e.g. an ISO sized 35 file will have a tip diameter of 35 hundredths of a millimetre or 0.35 mm. All ISO standard sized files are manufactured with a uniform '0.02' or two per cent taper. This means that the diameter of the file increases by 0.02 mm per millimetre increment away from the tip. ISO sized files are colour coded in a standard sequence (Table 5.2). Stainless steel hand files are generally manufactured in lengths 21 mm, 25 mm and 31 mm, although the cutting blades are 16 mm in length, regardless of the length of the files.

Stainless steel files—K-type files

Traditional K-files are manufactured by twisting a square blank of stainless steel alloy to produce sharp cutting flutes along the length of the file. K-files tend to be stiff, especially as the size increases. Many variations on the K-file design are available, including the K-Flex file (SybronEndo, Orange, CA, USA) and the K-Flexofile (Dentsply-Maillefer, Ballaigues, Switzerland). The K-Flex file has a rhomboid-shaped

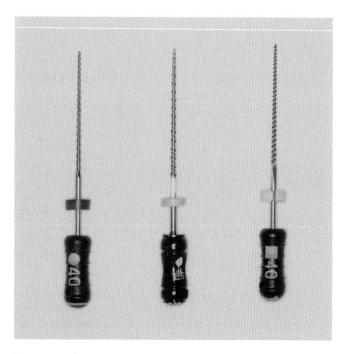

Figure 5.27 Selection of stainless steel files (from left to right): Hedström (SybronEndo, Orange, CA, USA), K-Flex and K-Flexofile (Dentsply-Maillefer, Ballaigues, Switzerland).

Table 5.2 ISO standard sized files and colour coding

Nominal size	Tip diameter (mm)	Colour
6	0.06	Pink
8	0.08	Grey
10	0.1	Purple
15	0.15	White
20	0.2	Yellow
25	0.25	Red
30	0.3	Blue
35	0.35	Green
40	0.4	Black
45	0.45	White
50	0.5	Yellow
55	0.55	Red
60	0.6	Blue
70	0.7	Green
80	0.8	Black

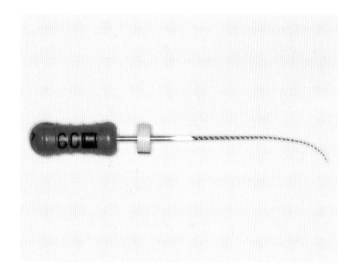

Figure 5.28 Pre-curved stainless steel file.

cross-section and is more flexible than traditional K-files. It has a cutting tip and is useful for negotiation of fine, calcified root canals. The K-Flexofile has a triangular cross-section and is very flexible compared with traditional K-files. It has a non-cutting tip, which is designed to reduce the risk of ledging and perforation.

Stainless steel files—Hedström files

Hedström files are manufactured by machining a round stainless steel blank to produce a continuous sequence of cones with sharp cutting edges and a cutting tip. Hedström files are used in a push-pull filing motion and they have an aggressive cutting action on withdrawal from the root canal. Rotational movements of greater than 30° should be avoided as Hedström files have a narrow core and are more susceptible to breakage than K-type files. They are useful for removing root canal filling materials during root canal retreatment.

Files for the negotiation of calcified root canals

Several files are available for initial negotiation of fine, calcified root canals (Fig. 5.29a,b). These are manufactured from a stiff steel alloy.

Nickel-titanium files

The development of nickel-titanium (NiTi) files has revolutionized root canal preparation (Fig 5.30). Nickel-titanium is a superelastic alloy, with a modulus of elasticity which is approximately one-fifth that of stainless steel. This property allows the alloy to undergo greater stresses than stainless steel, without breakage. It also exhibits 'shape memory' which means that it resists permanent deformation. Nickel-titanium files are able to withstand repeated cycles of compression and tension, which occur as a file is rotated in a curved root canal. The unique characteristics of NiTi alloy have made it possible to manufacture endodontic files which are larger in cross-section than stainless steel, with exceptional flexibility. This has led to the development of files, which have a greater taper (typically between four and eight per cent) than that of stainless steel files (which have a taper of two per cent). The advantage of NiTi files is that a tapered preparation is usually produced more quickly and with fewer files than with stainless steel hand files.

Many NiTi systems are available. Advances in metallurgy and file design continually lead to the development of new systems, e.g. TF files (SybronEndo, Orange, CA, USA) which are manufactured using a twisting process, and HyFlex CM (Coltene Whaledent, Altstätten, Switzerland) which have 'controlled memory' and do not exhibit the usual shape memory of NiTi files. It is generally claimed by the manufactures that new systems allow quicker root canal preparation with reduced risk of file breakage. Despite these claims, no system is necessarily superior to another. The majority of NiTi files are operated in a handpiece rotating at 150–500 rpm. Recently, NiTi files have been introduced which are operated in a reciprocating motion using a specialized endodontic motor, e.g. WaveOne (Dentsply-Maillefer, Ballaigues, Switzerland).

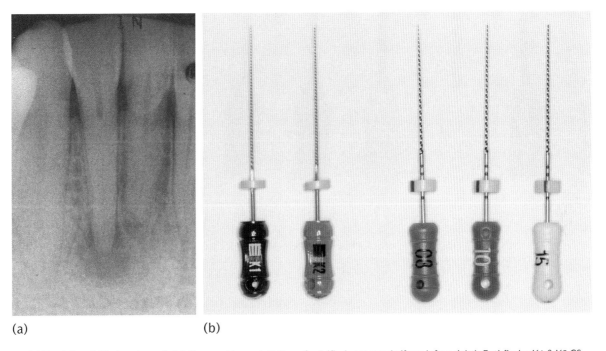

(a)   (b)

Figure 5.29 (a) Partially calcified root canal; (b) files used for negotiation of calcified root canals (from left to right): Pathfinder K1 & K2 CS (SybronEndo Orange, CA, USA) and C+ Files (Dentsply-Maillefer, Ballaigues, Switzerland).

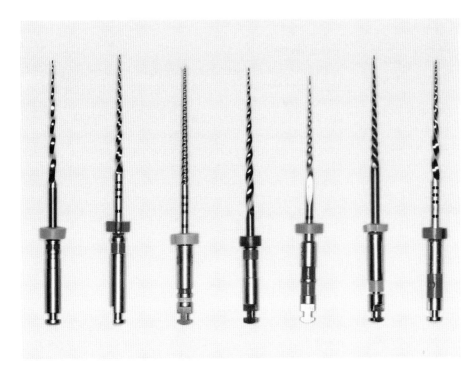

Figure 5.30 Selection of nickel-titanium (NiTi) machine driven files (from left to right): Race (FKG Dentaire, La Chaux-de-Fonds, Switzerland), ProTaper Universal (Dentsply-Maillefer, Ballaigues, Switzerland), K3 (SybronEndo, Orange, CA, USA), Revo-S (MicroMega, Besancon, France), TF (SybronEndo, Orange, CA, USA), HyFlex CM (Coltene Whaledent, Altstätten, Switzerland), WaveOne (Dentsply-Maillefer, Ballaigues, Switzerland).

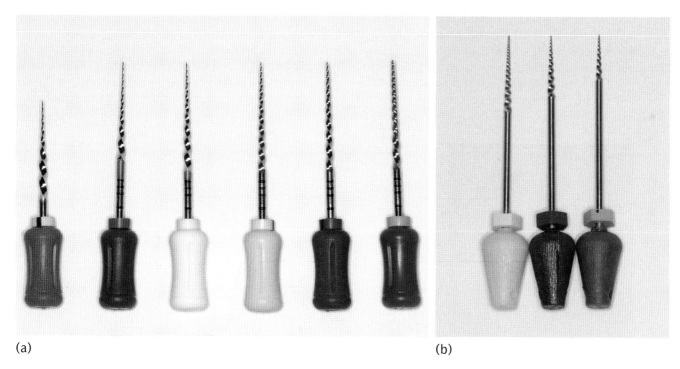

(a)   (b)

Figure 5.31 Nickel-titanium (NiTi) hand files: (a) ProTaper For Hand Use (Dentsply-Maillefer, Ballaigues, Switzerland) used in a balanced force technique; (b) GT Hand Files (Dentsply-Maillefer, Ballaigues, Switzerland) used in a reverse balanced force technique.

Nickel-titanium hand files are also available and these may be used when a motor is not available or when increased manual control is desired. Nickel-titanium files must be used with care and only after practice on training blocks or extracted teeth. If the correct procedures are not followed, NiTi files are liable to fracture.

Endodontic files may fracture due to:

- **Torsional stresses**: excessive torsional stresses are created when the tip of a file binds too tightly with the walls of the root canal while the file continues to rotate, leading to torsional fracture. Nickel-titanium files frequently have a tendency to 'screw in' to the root canal, which can lead to torsional fracture, especially if excessive speed or torque are applied. Files with a smaller cross-sectional area are more likely to fracture in this manner as they are less resistant to torsional failure.

- **Cyclic fatigue**: as the file rotates in a curved root canal, it undergoes repeated cycles of compression-tension, which eventually lead to fatigue of the alloy and file fracture. Files of a larger cross-sectional area are more likely to fracture by cyclic fatigue. This is because they are stiffer and undergo greater stresses when rotated in a curved root canal.

Chemical preparation

How is chemical preparation of the root canal system achieved?

Chemical preparation of the root canal system is achieved using irrigants which are delivered into the root canal system using side-vented

Instruments used for chemical preparation

Irrigation syringes and needles

Irrigant must be delivered into the root canals using side-vented needles. These increase the flow of irrigant out of the side of the needle and reduce the risk of irrigant extrusion into the periapical tissues. Luer-lock design syringes and needles should be used to ensure that the needle does not become detached during irrigation (Fig. 5.32).

Spiral fillers

Spiral fillers may be used to place intracanal medicaments or sealers into the root canal (Fig 5.33). They are available in a variety of sizes and are operated in a conventional slow speed handpiece. Care must be taken to ensure that the handpiece is rotating in a clockwise direction and that they are inserted passively into the root canal. If sufficient care is not taken, they can bind to the root canal walls and are liable to break. Caution must also be exercised to prevent forced extrusion of the medicament into the periapical tissues (e.g. inferior dental nerve, maxillary sinus) by ensuring the active instrument is not kept in the root canal for prolonged periods.

needles. The irrigant must be frequently agitated and replenished for effective cleaning and disinfection to be achieved. In addition, if the treatment is carried out over multiple visits (see Chapter 6), an interappointment medicament is used to further reduce the levels of microbes in the root canal system.

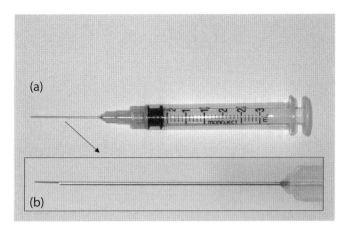

Figure 5.32 (a) Endodontic irrigation syringe and needle (Monoject, Covidien, Mansfield, MA, USA); (b) close-up view of side-venting needle.

The ideal irrigant should be:

- Antimicrobial;
- Cheap;
- Able to dissolve pulp tissue;
- Able to remove the smear layer;
- Easy to use;
- Have a long shelf-life;
- Have low surface tension;
- Non-staining;
- Non-cytotoxic/non-mutagenic;
- Compatible with dentine;
- Substantive (remain in the root canal for a sustained period);
- Tissue-friendly;
- Non-toxic;
- Non-corrosive to dental instruments.

Sodium hypochlorite

Sodium hypochlorite (NaOCl) fulfils most of the functions of an ideal irrigant (Fig. 5.34). It is a highly effective antimicrobial agent and it is able to dissolve residual pulp tissue and organic matter. Its antimicrobial properties are due to the action of free chlorine ions, which break down bacterial component proteins into constituent amino acids. A concentration of 0.5–3 per cent is generally recommended, although solutions of up to 5.25 per cent concentration are available. Studies have shown that lower concentrations are generally as bactericidal as higher concentrations. Higher concentrations have the benefit of increased tissue dissolving capacity but are also more irritant if any should be inadvertently be extruded into the periapical tissues ('hypochlorite accident'). Regular replenishment of NaOCl is necessary to maintain an effective level of free chlorine ions and agitation is recommended to maximize the dissolution of organic debris. A disadvantage of NaOCl is that it does not remove the smear layer.

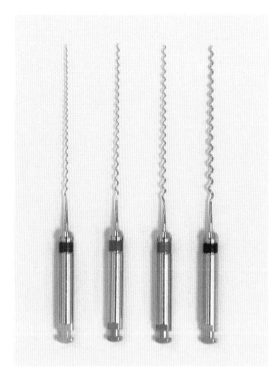

Figure 5.33 Selection of spiral fillers.

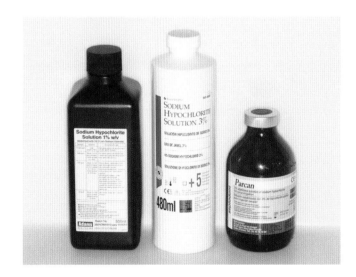

Figure 5.34 Sodium hypochlorite (NaOCl) solutions (left to right): Sodium hypochlorite solution 1% (Adams Healthcare, Leeds, UK); Sodium hypochlorite solution 3% (Henry Schein, Gillingham, UK); Parcan (Septodont, Saint-Maur-des-Fosses, France).

Ethylenediaminetetracetic acid

Ethylenediaminetetraacetic acid (EDTA) is a chelating agent, which removes the mineralized inorganic component of the dentine. It is used to remove the smear layer and aids the negotiation of calcified root canals. EDTA is usually used at a concentration of 17 per cent and is available as a solution (Fig. 5.35) or a paste (Fig. 5.36). EDTA pastes should be used sparingly as EDTA has an inhibitory effect on NaOCl

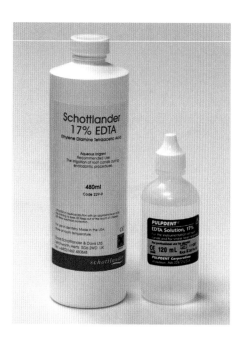

Figure 5.35 Ethylenediaminetetracetic acid (EDTA) solutions: Schottlander 17% EDTA (Schottlander, Letchworth, UK); Pulpdent EDTA Solution, 17% (Pulpdent, Watertown, MA, USA).

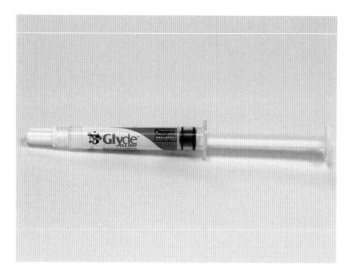

Figure 5.36 Ethylenediaminetetracetic acid (EDTA) paste: Glyde (Dentsply-Maillefer, Ballaigues, Switzerland).

and the carrier may adhere to the root canal walls, preventing effective disinfection by NaCOl.

What is the smear layer and what is its relevance to endodontic treatment?

The smear layer is an amorphous film of organic and inorganic material generated from instruments contacting the root canal walls. It is composed of a superficial layer on the root canal surface (1–2 µm) and plugs penetrating up to 40 µm into the dentinal tubules. It is generally recommended that the smear layer should be removed (Table 5.3).

Alternative irrigants

Chlorhexidine gluconate

Chlorhexidine gluconate has a high degree of antimicrobial activity and has been suggested as an irrigant in root canal retreatment (Fig. 5.37). This is because *ex-vivo* studies have demonstrated that it is effective against certain microbes (e.g. *Enterococcus faecalis*) that are more commonly found in retreatment cases. Chlorhexidine gluconate solution of 0.12–0.2 per cent may be used, although a solution of 2 per cent concentration is available for use as a root canal irrigant. A disadvantage of chlorhexidine gluconate is that it is unable to dissolve organic or inorganic tissue, so it is generally not considered to be such an effective irrigant as NaCOl. However, it is useful in situations where NaCOl is unsuitable to use, such as in patients who have an allergy to household bleach. Chlorhexidine gluconate solution forms a toxic precipitate when combined with NaCOl, so if both irrigants are used, the root canal system should be rinsed with saline and dried with paper

Table 5.3 Benefits of smear layer removal

- The smear layer harbours microbes and may also act as nutriment for microbes
- The smear layer may act as a barrier to irrigant and medicament penetration
- The smear layer may influence the quality of the bond obtainable with root canal sealers
- If the smear layer disintegrates after the root filling has been completed, it will affect the seal of the root canal filling material

points when switching between the two irrigants. Evidence is emerging that when chlorhexidine gluconate is used in combination with NaCOl, success rates for root canal treatment are reduced.

Iodine compounds

Iodine potassium iodide is an effective antimicrobial agent and may be used as a final root canal irrigant in retreatment cases. However, it has the potential to induce an allergic reaction in some patients and causes staining of dentine.

Why is it necessary to agitate the irrigant?

During preparation, the irrigant may be agitated using a small (size 10/15) file. At the end of root canal preparation and before filling, it is recommended that the irrigant is agitated by moving a well-fitting GP point vigorously up and down in the root canal or by passive ultrasonic irrigation.

The aims of irrigant agitation are to:

- Promote irrigant exchange apically;
- Circulate the irrigant to the parts of the root canal system that are not touched by mechanical preparation techniques;
- Stir up debris, therefore reducing blockages;

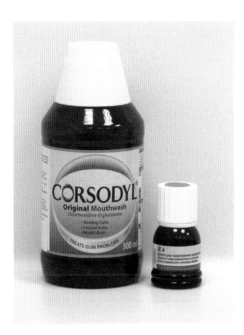

Figure 5.37 Chlorhexidine gluconate solutions (left to right): Corsodyl (GlaxoSmithKline Consumer Healthcare, Brentford, UK) and R4 (Septodont, Saint-Maur-des-Fosses, France).

- Dislodge microbial biofilm from the root canal walls;
- Encourage dissolution of organic matter;
- Aid smear layer removal.

Files may be made to vibrate at very high frequencies (2–30 kHz), by generating acoustic energy which can be transmitted to the file as mechanical energy. This is known as passive ultrasonic irrigation. When files are ultrasonically activated in the root canal, the irrigant immediately surrounding the file becomes turbulent (acoustic microstreaming) and the temperature of the irrigant increases, resulting in enhanced debridement and disinfection of the root canal. In order for acoustic microstreaming to take place, the root canal has to be wide enough to allow unrestricted movement of the ultrasonic file; otherwise it will become dampened against the root canal wall and may lead to the creation of aberrations. For example, an activated size 15 file will only be effective in a root canal that has been prepared up to a size 40. Ultrasonic irrigation should therefore only be attempted after the root canal has been prepared completely.

What is the purpose of intracanal medicaments?

Medicaments are usually placed into root canals between the preparation and root canal filling visits, i.e. interappointment medicament. This may be planned or carried out when there is insufficient time to complete treatment in one visit.

Actions of intracanal medicaments:

- Medicaments inhibit the proliferation of microbes between visits;
- Medicaments further reduce the numbers of microbes in the root canal system;
- Degradation of residual necrotic tissue;
- Control of apical serous exudate;
- Long-lasting antimicrobial effect;
- Killing of microbes in fins, isthmuses, and ramifications;
- Medicaments allow symptoms (e.g. pain, swelling, or a discharging sinus) to settle prior to root canal filling and restoration.

Calcium hydroxide

Calcium hydroxide is the intracanal medicament of choice (Fig. 5.38 and Table 5.4). Calcium hydroxide is available commercially as ready-mixed pastes or as pure powder which can be mixed with water or saline to produce a paste of the desired consistency.

Ledermix paste

Ledermix paste (Blackwell Supplies, Gillingham, UK) contains a steroid (triamcinolone acetonide) and an antibiotic (demeclocycline hydrochloride) (Fig. 5.39). Its main use is in the treatment of the pulpitic tooth. The steroid is thought to be of value in reducing pulpal inflammation and pain. It is however of limited use as an interappointment medicament in non-vital teeth as is has limited antimicrobial activity. Furthermore, its use may give rise to bacterial resistance.

Iodine compounds

Iodine compounds have been demonstrated in ex-vivo studies to be effective against some strains of bacteria that are resistant to calcium

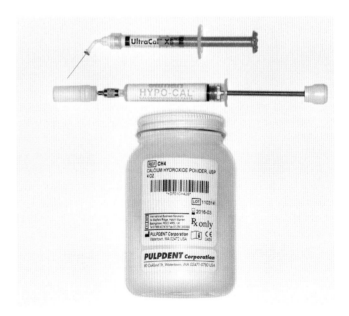

Figure 5.38 Calcium hydroxide paste: UltraCal XS syringe and NaviTip (Ultradent, South Jordan, UT, USA), Hypo-cal (Ellman, Oceanside, NY, USA), and calcium hydroxide powder (Pulpdent, Watertown, MA, USA).

Table 5.4 Properties of calcium hydroxide

Properties of calcium hydroxide	Actions	Potential disadvantages
Limited solubility	Calcium hydroxide physically prevents growth of microbes and has been demonstrated to substantially reduce the numbers of cultivable bacteria in the root canal	Some bacteria, notably *Enterococcus faecalis*, have been found to be resistant
High pH (12)	Degrades residual pulpal tissue (synergistic action with sodium hypochlorite)	It may not always be possible to remove all calcium hydroxide from the root canal, which may result in a suboptimal root canal filling
Broad spectrum antimicrobial agent	Induction of apical hard barrier in teeth with wide open apices	Calcium hydroxide weakens dentine if left in the root canal for extended periods
Antimicrobial action sustained over a long duration	Control of serous exudate	

hydroxide. As an intracanal medicament, they are commercially available as Vitapex (Neo Dental, Federal Way, WA, USA) and Metapex (Meta Dental, Glendale, NY, USA), which are pastes containing calcium hydroxide and iodoform. These are inappropriate for use in patients who are allergic to iodine-containing compounds.

Phenolic preparations

Phenolic compounds, e.g. paramonochlorophenol, used to be the most commonly used medicaments. Their use has fallen out of favour in recent years as their antibacterial effects are short-lived; they are volatile compounds which are able to diffuse through the temporary filling material and are irritant to the periapical tissues. Their use has been superseded by calcium hydroxide, which has been demonstrated to be a more effective and long-lasting antimicrobial agent.

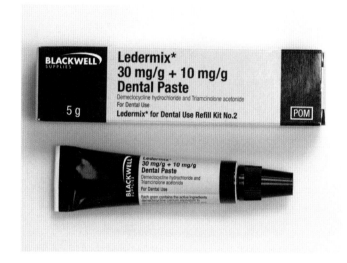

Figure 5.39 Ledermix paste (Blackwell Supplies, Gillingham, UK).

Why is a good temporary restoration required?

Before removing the rubber dam and discharging the patient, a well-adapted and durable temporary restoration must be placed in the access cavity to provide a good coronal seal and to support the remaining coronal tooth structure. Failure to provide a good temporary restoration will result in contamination of the root canals by microbes from the oral environment, which in some cases may subsequently be extremely difficult to eliminate. The access cavity should have suitable resistance form to prevent the displacement of the temporary restoration. Reinforced zinc oxide eugenol dressing, e.g. IRM (Dentsply DeTrey, Konstanz, Germany), or glass ionomer cement, e.g. Fuji IX (GC Corporation, Tokyo, Japan), are both ideal temporary restoration materials (Fig. 5.40). Premixed temporary filling materials are not recommended as they are prone to wear away or wash out of the access cavity.

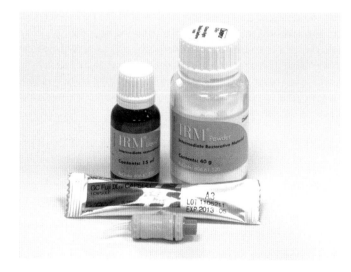

Figure 5.40 Materials that may be used as temporary restorations: IRM (Dentsply DeTrey, Konstanz, Germany) and Fuji IX (GC Corporation, Tokyo, Japan).

Foundations of clinical practice

The remainder of this chapter covers the practical aspects of root canal preparation. Although individual methods of preparation may vary, the principles remain the same. Root canal treatment must only be carried out with patient's consent after a thorough clinical examination (including special investigations), diagnosis, and discussion of treatment options has been carried out.

Pretreatment assessment and preparation of the tooth

Before starting root canal treatment, a thorough clinical and radiographic assessment of the tooth needs to be made.

Clinical assessment

Clinically, an assessment needs to be made of:

- Existing restoration(s);
- Restorability of the tooth;
- Tooth angulation;
- Tooth rotation;
- Positions of the cemento–enamel junction and furcation.

Prior to access cavity preparation, restorations must be carefully assessed. Teeth that require endodontic treatment are frequently heavily restored and may have associated carious lesions. Leaking restorations (Fig. 5.41) and caries must be removed to avoid the introduction of carious dentine and microbes into the root canals.

Full coverage restorations may have defective margins and may be undermined by caries, which may not be easily detected clinically or radiographically. Furthermore, the presence of full coverage restorations will often obscure anatomical landmarks and mask the true orientation of the tooth, which may result in removal of excessive amounts of sound dentine (Fig. 5.42) when attempting to locate the root canals; this may result in iatrogenic perforation and/or rendering the tooth unrestorable. Cuspal coverage restorations can also limit visibility in the floor of the access cavity, causing difficulties in locating the root canal entrance(s).

Ideally, existing restorations should be removed from the tooth under investigation prior to embarking on root canal treatment. This enables a full assessment of the structure and integrity of the tooth, and may reveal the presence of cracks (Fig. 5.43a,b), which could influence the prognosis of the tooth and the design of the subsequent restoration. The patient must be fully aware of the procedure and have given their consent to the exploratory work.

However, if the tooth has a cuspal coverage restoration that was provided recently, or the clinician is confident that the margins are sound, access may be made through the restoration. When access is made through a cuspal coverage restoration, ceramic fracture may occur or caries may be discovered beneath the restoration. The patient should always be warned before treatment that a new restoration might be required afterwards.

Before commencing root canal treatment, unsupported/cracked cusps may be reduced in height, and/or an orthodontic band may be cemented to reduce the chances of the tooth fracturing. A provisional restoration may be required to facilitate rubber dam placement and to provide a reservoir for irrigants.

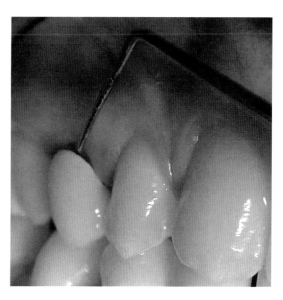

Figure 5.41 Clinical evidence of leakage around restoration margin, this crown should be removed to allow the restorability of the tooth to be assessed before embarking on endodontic treatment.

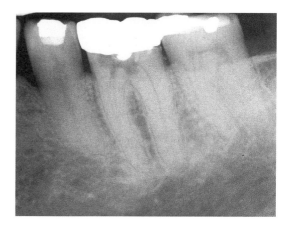

Figure 5.42 Radiographic evidence of excessive removal of dentine when attempting to locate the root canals. More sound tooth tissue may have been retained had the existing restoration been removed before embarking on endodontic treatment.

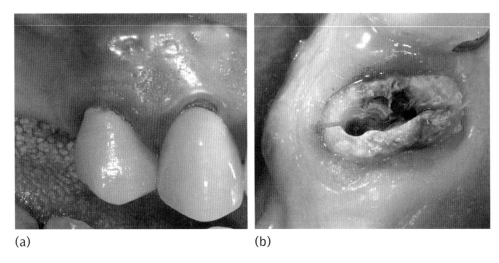

(a)   (b)

Figure 5.43 Removal of the existing restoration (a) revealed a catastrophic crack rendering the tooth unrestorable. (b).

Radiographic assessment

A clear, undistorted periapical radiograph of the tooth to be treated should always be available prior to commencing treatment. The criteria for success when taking radiographs are as follows:

- Use a paralleling technique (use a film or digital sensor holder and beam aiming device);
- Create minimal geometric distortion (elongation or foreshortening) by not bending of the film or incorrect patient and/or X ray tube positioning;
- The complete tooth should be visible, including ≥ 3 mm of the periapical bone;
- Employ the correct procedures for exposure, developing, mounting, and labelling of radiographs.

An assessment of the periapical radiograph along with any relevant bitewing radiographs should be made to assess:

- The position, size, and shape of the pulp chamber and the presence or absence of pulp horns;
- The degree of calcification of the pulp chamber and the root canals;
- The position of the root canal entrances;
- The morphology and curvature of the root canals;
- The estimated working length of root canals.

A bur mounted in a handpiece may be held up against the preoperative radiograph to estimate the depth of the floor of the pulp chamber.

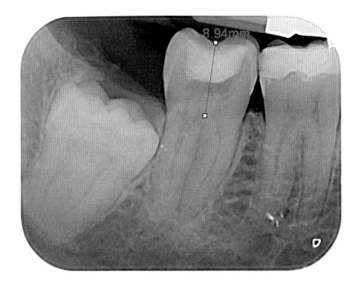

Figure 5.44 Estimating the depth of the pulp chamber using computer software. Note the calcifications in the pulp chamber.

If the floor of the pulp chamber is obscured by a metallic restoration, the furcation may be used as a reference point to estimate the position of the pulp chamber. If digital radiographs are employed, the software that is used to view the images must be calibrated to enable the lengths of the root canals and the depth of the pulp chamber to be estimated (Fig. 5.44).

Access cavity preparation

The shape of the access cavity is determined by the number and location of the root canals. Initial penetration into the pulp chamber should be made through the crown of the tooth at a point where the floor and the pulp chamber are at their furthest distance apart. This is frequently over the pulp horns. A tungsten carbide cross cut fissure bur is ideal for initial access cavity preparation, especially if cutting through metallic restorations. If access is made through metal-ceramic or all-ceramic crowns, a diamond bur should be used to efficiently cut through the ceramic.

When initial penetration is made, the bur will be felt to drop into the pulp chamber (Fig. 5.45). At this point, a non-end cutting bur (e.g. Endo-Z bur; Dentsply-Maillefer, Ballaigues, Switzerland) can be used to completely remove the roof of the pulp chamber and to refine the sides of the access cavity without damaging the floor of the pulp chamber (Fig. 5.46). In cases where extensive calcification of the pulp chamber has occurred, a drop into the pulp chamber will not be felt. In these cases, extreme care must be taken during access cavity preparation not to create a perforation. It is important to remove the entire roof of the pulp chamber so that all coronal pulp tissue may be removed (Fig. 5.47). The walls of the access cavity should be probed to ensure that the entire

roof of the pulp chamber has been removed and there are no lips of dentine remaining (Fig. 5.48). Care should be taken to be as conservative of tooth substance as possible (Fig. 5.49) and avoid damaging the floor of the pulp chamber (Fig. 5.50).

The objectives of access cavity preparation are to:

- Remove the entire roof of the pulp chamber so that all coronal pulp tissue may be removed (*note*: anterior teeth do not have a pulpal floor—the pulp chamber merges into the root canal);
- Allow visualization of root canal entrances (Fig. 5.51);
- Produce a smooth-walled preparation with no overhangs of dentine;
- Allow unimpeded straight-line access of instruments into the coronal third of each root canal(s).

Location of root canal entrances

An endodontic explorer is used to probe the floor of the pulp chamber to locate the root canal entrances. Good lighting is essential and the use of dental loupes or a dental operating microscope is recommended. The floor of the pulp chamber is darker and greyer in colour than the walls of the pulp chamber (Fig. 5.51). Developmental lines may be seen running across the floor of the pulp chamber 'mapping out' the location of the entrance of root canal(s). In general root canals tend to be symmetrically placed. Therefore, if a single root canal is found, but it is situated towards the buccal or lingual side of the tooth, another root canal is likely to be present.

Deposits of tertiary dentine may obscure the root canal entrances and cause narrowing or calcification of the coronal portion of the

root canals. Tertiary dentine is more white and opaque than primary and secondary dentine and can provide a clue to the location of root canal entrances. Removal should be undertaken judiciously using long neck burs, gooseneck burs, or specialized endodontic ultrasonic tips in a piezo-electric ultrasonic unit. Indiscriminate and excessive dentine removal may lead to perforations laterally or into the furcation, which ultimately compromise the future prognosis of the tooth. If difficulty is encountered when attempting to locate the entrances to root canals, a radiograph should be taken to check the location of the root canals in relation to the access cavity already prepared. In especially difficult cases, referral to a specialist in endodontics should be considered.

Creating straight-line access

Once the root canal entrances have been identified, it is often necessary to modify the shape of the root canal entrances and the access cavity to allow unimpeded access for files into the root canals (straight-line

access). This may be achieved using a variety of instruments, including Gates Glidden drills, NiTi orifice shapers and non-end cutting burs.

Techniques used for the manipulation of hand files

Once straight-line access has been established, the root canal(s) can be instrumented. Stainless steel hand files are used for initial negotiation. Hand files may be manipulated using several different techniques to negotiate and shape the root canal system.

Watch-winding technique

This is a useful technique for initial negotiation of the coronal and apical portions of the root canal. The technique involves gently rotating a small hand file alternately clockwise and anticlockwise, approximately 30°, whilst maintaining gentle apical pressure. When progression becomes difficult, the file should be withdrawn to remove

debris. The use of copious irrigant and lubrication facilitates the progression of files apically.

Balanced-force technique

The balanced-force technique allows controlled manipulation of hand files whilst maintaining a centred preparation and reducing the incidence of procedural errors (Fig. 5.52a,b, and c). The technique is useful during initial root canal negotiation, coronal flaring, and apical preparation. It works well with stainless steel K-Flexofiles and hand NiTi ProTaper files. If hand GT (Dentsply-Maillefer, Ballaigues, Switzerland) files are used, a reverse balanced-force technique is

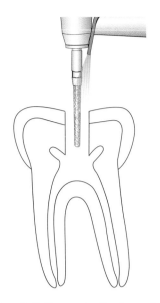

Figure 5.45 Bur penetrating the roof of the pulp chamber.

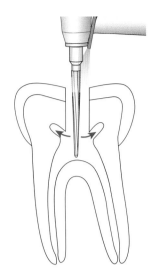

Figure 5.46 Non-end cutting bur removing remainder of the roof of the pulp chamber.

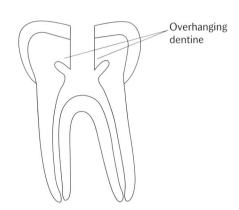

Figure 5.47 Inadequate access cavity with incomplete removal of the roof of the pulp chamber.

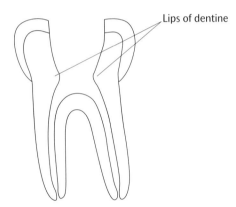

Figure 5.48 Inadequate access cavity with lip of dentine remaining.

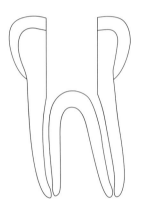

Figure 5.49 Ideal access cavity preparation.

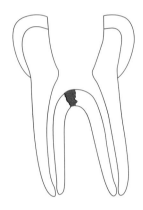

Figure 5.50 Perforation of the pulp chamber floor.

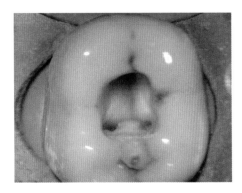

Figure 5.51 Access cavity allowing visualization of the root canals.

(a) Engage dentine: Rotate a quarter turn clockwise

(b) Cut dentine: Rotate a half turn anticlockwise with firm apical pressure

(c) Remove dentine: Rotate a quarter turn clockwise

Figure 5.52 Balanced-force technique: (a) quarter turn clockwise; (b) half turn anticlockwise whilst maintaining apical pressure; (c) quarter turn clockwise and withdraw.

used (i.e. the files are rotated in an anticlockwise direction first). This technique must not be carried out with Hedström files as it will result in file fracture. The balanced-force technique is carried out as follows:

- The file is inserted into the root canal until resistance is felt and rotated a quarter of a turn clockwise to engage dentine in the flutes of the file;
- The file is then rotated anticlockwise for a half turn whilst maintaining apical pressure (to prevent the file from reversing out of the root canal). This action cuts dentine from the walls of the root canal and a characteristic 'click' may be heard and felt;
- A further clockwise rotation through a quarter turn collects debris on the flutes of the file before withdrawing from the root canal;

- The first two steps may be repeated twice before withdrawing the file;
- Ensure all debris is removed from the file and check for signs of file distortion before reinsertion;
- Files should not be pre-curved when the balanced force technique is used.

Push-pull technique

The push-pull filing technique is used to plane the walls of the root canal. The file is moved up and down in the root canal in small increments (1–3 mm). This technique is ideal for use with Hedström files, but it may also be carried out with K-type files. It is a useful technique for smoothing ledges in root canals once they have been successfully bypassed.

Initial negotiation

Initial root canal negotiation is carried out with an ISO size 10 or 15 file, which should be gently worked apically using a watch-winding motion to ensure that the coronal portion of the root canal is negotiable. At this stage, it is not necessary to negotiate the root canal to the apex. The pulp chamber should be flooded with NaCOI to facilitate negotiation and to avoid the creation of blockages. EDTA lubricant can also be used to aid initial negotiation. The initial file should fit fairly passively in the root canal and should never be forced apically as this can result in procedural errors. If the root canal is fine or tortuous, an ISO size 06 or

08 file should be used. Files are available which are designed specifically for the initial negotiation of calcified root canals. The ease with which the initial file passes down the root canal can give an indication of the presence of curvatures that are not visible radiographically, i.e. curvatures in the bucco–lingual plane, and the joining or separation of root canals. Files should be examined upon removal from the root canal for the presence of bends which give an indication of the root canal shape. Sequentially larger files, up to ISO size 20, should be used to create a 'glide path' in the coronal portion of the root canal.

Coronal flaring

Coronal flaring is the next stage in root canal instrumentation. The coronal third to half of the root canal is flared to produce a gradual taper, which is widest at the root canal entrances.

- Coronal flaring may be achieved using a combination of stainless steel hand files, Gates Glidden drills and/or NiTi hand/machine driven files.
- Sequentially smaller instruments are used as progress is made from the coronal to the apical third of the root canal—each instrument creates space for smaller sized instruments to advance further down the root canal.
- Gates Glidden drills must be used with great care. They can only be used in the straight part of the root canal so their depth of penetration is limited by the curvature of the root canal. Sizes 2 and 3 Gates Glidden drills are appropriate for use in most root canals. Size 1 Gates

Glidden drills are very prone to breakage and sizes 4 and above are only suitable for use in larger root canals, as they are liable to cause strip perforations if used inappropriately.

- Nickel-titanium files are more flexible and can be used beyond the root canal curvature; they also allow more rapid instrumentation of the root canal than Gates Glidden drills. Some systems have specific files (orifice shapers) which are designed for coronal flaring, whilst in other systems, files of decreasing taper or diameter are employed in a crown-down approach.
- After removal of each file from the root canal, the flutes should be inspected for debris and cleaned using a sponge or gauze. The root canal should be irrigated and recapitulated with an ISO size 10 or 15 hand file to prevent blockage of the root canal by debris beyond the level of instrumentation.

Apical negotiation

When coronal flaring has been completed, the full length of the root canal may be negotiated in a similar manner to that used for initial negotiation. If the root canal is narrow, small sized hand files should

be used to negotiate the root canal to the full length, using a gentle watch-winding motion. The apical portions of root canals frequently have sharp curvatures which are challenging to negotiate. Files should never be forced as this leads to procedural errors such as ledges and perforations. If the root canal is curved, small sized stainless steel files can be pre-curved to negotiate the curvature (Fig. 5.28). The location and severity of such curvatures should be noted, as they influence the preparation of the apical portion of the root canal. Table 5.5 gives tips on preparing curved root canals.

Table 5.5 Tips on preparing curved root canals

- Use a coronal-to-apical preparation technique (e.g. Crown-down and modified double flare techniques)
- Pre-curve files to match the curvature of the root canal
- Use more flexible files: small ISO size files or nickel-titanium (NiTi) files
- Keep the preparation small
- Preferentially file the outer walls of the root canal, i.e. away from the furcation wall (anti-curvature filing)

Working length determination

The working length may be determined by taking a diagnostic (working length) radiograph or by using an EAL. Electronic apex locators are generally reliable, but if any doubt exists about the accuracy of the reading given, a diagnostic radiograph should be taken.

Radiograph technique

Estimate the root canal length from an accurate preoperative radiograph;

- Place a file into the root canal to the estimated working length (Fig. 5.53a);
- A minimum file size of 10 should be used, (ideally size 15), as smaller files may not be clearly visible radiographically. In a large root canal, use the first size that binds in the apical region. This is known as the diagnostic file;
- Identify a reproducible coronal reference point (e.g. a cusp tip or incisal edge) and ensure that the silicone stop on the file is contacting the reference point before and after taking the radiograph;
- Take a radiograph using a paralleling technique using an endodontic radiograph holder (Fig. 5.53b);
- The complete tooth should be visible and ideally ≥ 3 mm of the surrounding periapical tissues (Fig. 5.53c);
- If the radiograph reveals that the file is within 2 mm of the radiographic apex, any necessary adjustments to the length of the file can be made and instrumentation may be continued. If the file is more than 2 mm from the correct length, the length should be adjusted and another radiograph taken to confirm the correct working length;
- If two root canals are in the same plane, e.g. two mesial root canals in a mandibular molar, they may be distinguished radiographically by using a Hedström file in one of the root canals and a K-type file in the other. The buccal object rule may be used to 'separate' the root canals radiographically; the tube is angulated mesially or distally by approximately 10°.

Electronic apex locator technique

Estimate the root canal length from an accurate preoperative radiograph;

- Ensure there is no excess fluid (irrigant, blood, or pus) in the pulp chamber or coronal half of the root canal;
- Place the lip hook on the patient's lip (Fig. 5.54a);
- Place a small file (e.g. ISO size 10 or 15) into the root canal and attach the file clip (Fig. 5.54b);
- 'Watch-wind' the file gently apically until the display on the EAL indicates that the file tip is at the apical foramen (known as the 'zero reading' and displayed as either 'APEX', 'red segment', or '0') (Fig. 5.54c);
- Ensure that the silicone stop on the file is contacting a reproducible coronal reference point before removing the file;
- On removing the file, measure the recorded length;
- Determine the working length by subtracting 0.5–1.0 mm from the recorded 'zero reading'.

Care must be taken when using apex locators to ensure that the reading is as accurate as possible.

The following factors may cause unreliable readings:

- Metallic restorations: ensure that the file does not contact metallic restorations or a short circuit will occur;
- Pulp remnants, especially at the root canal apices;
- Low batteries;
- Leaking rubber dam;
- Wide apical foramen: in teeth with large apices, a larger file may be required to obtain an accurate reading;
- Excessive fluid in root canal.

Apical preparation

After the working length has been determined, apical preparation of the root canal is completed using stainless steel hand files alone, or a combination of NiTi (machine-driven or hand) files and stainless steel files.

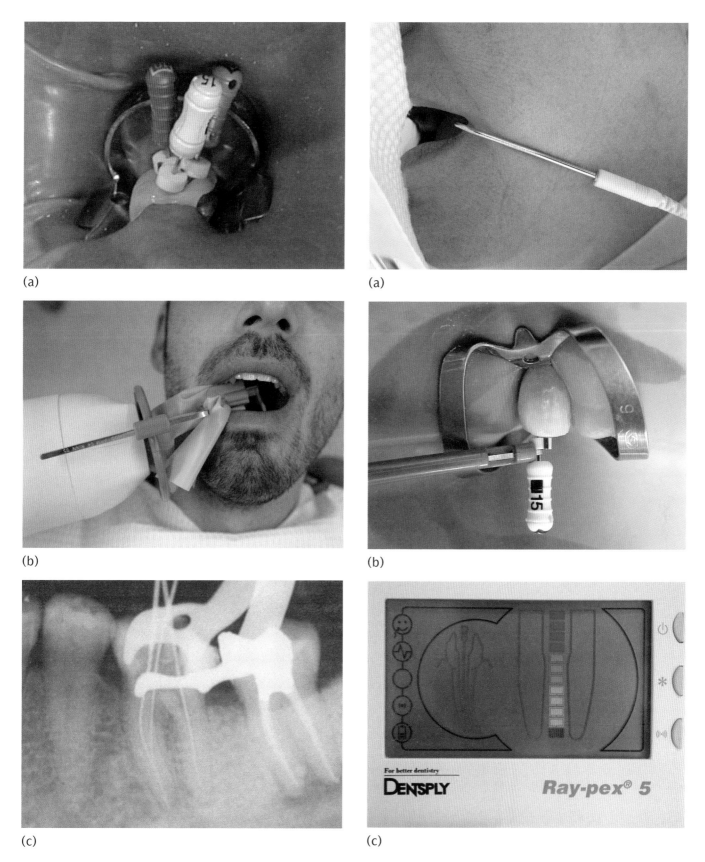

Figure 5.53 Working length determination using the radiograph technique: (a) files in the root canals at estimated working length; (b) endo holder in use; (c) working length radiograph.

Figure 5.54 Working length determination using the electronic apex locator (EAL) technique: (a) lip hook resting on patient's lip; (b) file clip in contact with file; (c) 'zero reading' on display.

Crown-down technique

After coronal flaring and working length determination, the remainder of the root canal is prepared, and a taper achieved by using files in a sequence of larger to smaller sizes, progressing apically. Once the working length is reached, the sequence is repeated using larger files until a file of the desired size for the apical preparation reaches the working length. This technique was originally described for use with stainless steel hand files but is now routinely carried out using NiTi files (Fig. 5.55).

Modified double flare technique

The modified double flare technique refers to the preparation of the coronal portion of the root canal to a taper, as already described, followed by apical preparation using stainless steel hand files. Apical preparation is carried out in two stages:

- Apical enlargement;
- Creation of apical taper (or deep shaping).

Apical enlargement

- The diameter of the apical portion of the root canal should be gauged by inserting ISO hand files passively to the established working length until a file binds at the working length.
- The smallest acceptable apical preparation is usually equivalent to an ISO size 25 file.
- Files are used in sequentially larger sizes at the established working length to increase the size of the apical preparation (Fig. 5.56a).
- The largest file used to the full working length is the master apical file (MAF). This size is dependent on the original size and curvature of

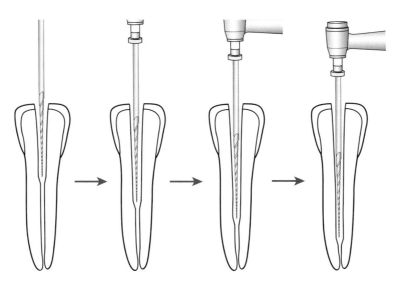

Figure 5.55 Apical preparation using a crown-down technique.

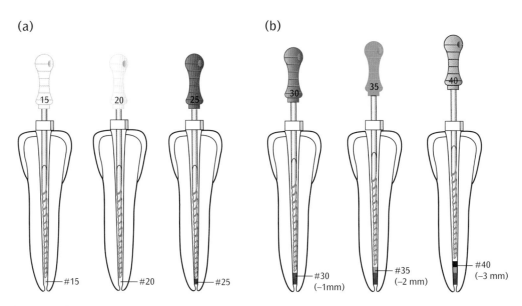

Figure 5.56 Modified double flare technique: (a) apical enlargement and (b) apical taper.

Table 5.6 Tips for using machine-driven nickel-titanium (NiTi) files

- Practice on endodontic training blocks and extracted teeth.
- Use with a dedicated endodontic electric motor and speed reducing handpiece with torque control.
- Refer to the manufacturer's protocol for speed and torque for each file used.
- Ensure that straight-line access has been established before introducing NiTi files into the root canals to avoid placing unnecessary stresses on the files.
- NiTi files are an adjunct to, rather than a replacement for, stainless steel hand files. It is essential to ensure that a glide path is achieved with at least a size 15 hand file prior to the introduction of rotary NiTi files to avoid procedural accidents and to minimize the incidence of file breakage.
- The file must be rotating before entering and on removal from the root canal.
- A light touch is required (a similar amount of pressure as applied when writing with a lead pencil).
- Use a pecking motion—never force the file or keep at the same point within a root canal.
- The root canal(s) and pulp chamber should be flooded with irrigant to reduce friction and to prevent blockages and file breakage.
- Check files upon removal from the root canal—discard files with signs of deformation.
- Great care must be exercised when instrumenting root canals with severe curvatures.

the root canal. For example, a central incisor in a young patient may have an ISO size 50 MAF or larger, whilst a curved, partially calcified mesio-buccal root canal of a maxillary molar may have an ISO size 25 MAF.

- Frequent irrigation is essential.

Apical taper (or deep shaping)

- Files of increasing size are used sequentially in an apical to coronal approach, stepping back in 1 mm increments. This creates an apical taper and blends the apical preparation with the coronal flare (Fig. 5.56b).
- After each file is used, the root canal should be irrigated and recapitulated with the master apical file to the full working length to ensure that the root canal does not become blocked with debris.
- After the apical taper has been created, the root canal should taper smoothly from the entrance of the root canal coronally to the apical terminus of the preparation.

Apical preparation with nickel-titanium files

Generally, when NiTi files are used, the coronal flaring and apical preparation are carried out using a NiTi file system according to the manufacturer's protocol (Table 5.6). Some NiTi systems are used

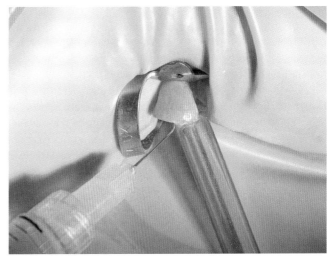

(a)

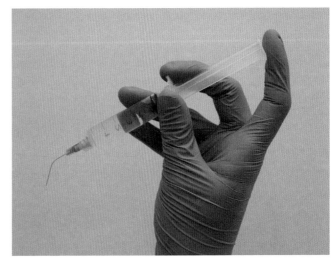

(b)

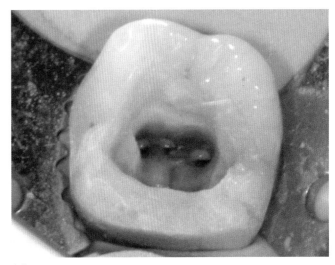

(c)

Figure 5.57 (a) Root canal being irrigated; (b) a forefinger should be used to apply gentle pressure to the plunger; (c) sodium hypochlorite (NaCOl) in root canals, note three mesial root canals associated with this mandibular molar.

in a crown-down approach, either using files of the same taper with decreasing tip size or using files of the same tip size with decreasing taper. Some systems use a combination of the two. In other NiTi systems files of varying taper and tip size are sequentially taken to the full working length.

Before using NiTi files in the apical portion of the root canal, a glide path should be created using a size 15–20 stainless steel hand file. The apex should be gauged using hand files to determine the diameter of the root canal at the full working length. Once the apex has been gauged, NiTi instrumentation may be completed until a NiTi file of suitable diameter and taper reaches the full working length. Table 5.6 gives tips for using machine-driven NiTi files.

Patency filing

Regardless of the technique used for apical preparation, patency should be maintained throughout the procedure. A small hand file (ISO size 10 or smaller) should be inserted 0.5–1.0 mm through the apical constriction to prevent blockage of the apical portion of the root canal with infected debris. The file should not be inserted any further through the constriction than 0.5–1.0 mm to avoid pushing infected debris into the periapical tissues.

Procedures for chemical preparation

Irrigation

The root canal system should be irrigated at every stage of the preparation with an antimicrobial solution. The irrigant of choice is a 0.5–3.0 per cent solution of NaOCl. Whilst frequent irrigation may seem tedious and time-consuming, it is essential for the removal of microbes and debris. If insufficiently irrigated, the root canal can easily become blocked with dentine chips, which may make further instrumentation very difficult and lead to procedural errors such as ledges and perforations (Fig. 5.57a,b,c).

The criteria for successful irrigation are as follows:

- Ensure that the rubber dam seals the working area;
- Use a Luer-Lock syringe and a side-vented needle;
- Apply a rubber/silicone stop to the needle to measure the depth of penetration, which should be at least 2 mm short of the working length;
- Apply gentle pressure to the plunger of the syringe, using a forefinger rather than a thumb;
- Irrigate frequently, ideally after each file is withdrawn from the root canal, and always ensure that there is a reservoir of irrigant in the pulp chamber.

Great care must be taken to avoid extrusion of irrigant into the apical tissues. Extrusion should be avoided if the criteria listed above are followed. Table 5.7 lists the symptoms of NaOCl extrusion (hypochlorite accident) and the action required.

Table 5.7 Symptoms and management of sodium hypochlorite (NaOCl) accident

Symptoms	Management
Acute severe pain and swelling	• Be calm • Reassure the patient and advise them of what has happened • Advise the patient that the swelling may take up to a week to reduce fully • Prescribe analgesics and antibiotics
Profuse bleeding from root canal	• Irrigate the root canal with saline, dry and apply a temporary dressing
Taste of chlorine and throat irritation (if NaOCl is extruded into the maxillary sinus)	• Ask the patient to drink water or milk
Bruising or ecchymosis of the skin or mucosa	• Advise the patient to apply a cold compress • Advise the patient that bruising may take up to a week to reduce fully
Longer term paraesthesia or anaesthesia	• Refer to hospital and inform patient
Symptoms starting to resolve	• Recall after 1–3 days to review symptoms • Determine why the accident occurred • Once the patient is symptom-free, complete the root canal treatment or refer to a specialist in endodontics

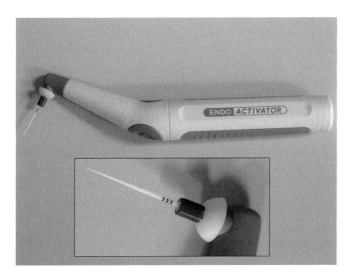

Figure 5.58 EndoActivator system (Dentsply Tulsa Dental Specialties, Tulsa, OK, USA).

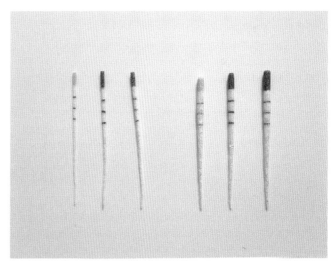

Figure 5.60 Selection of paper points: standard sized (left) and tapered (right).

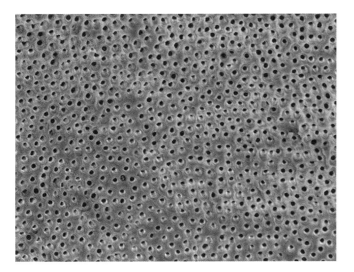

Figure 5.59 Scanning electron micrograph of the root canal wall following smear layer removal. Note the 'clean' surface and patent dentine tubules.

Passive ultrasonic irrigation (PUI) is a more effective means of irrigant agitation. This involves the introduction of a small (usually size 15) ultrasonically activated file into the root canal. The file should be placed passively into the root canal without touching the root canal walls. The activation of the file warms the irrigant and causes acoustic microstreaming, which dislodges organic debris and microbial biofilm, and aids penetration of the irrigant into the parts of the root canal that are inaccessible to mechanical preparation. Another means of irrigant agitation is sonic irrigation which involves the introduction of a sonically activated single-use polymer tip into the root canal (Fig. 5.58).

Smear layer removal

The smear layer is removed by irrigating with EDTA solution, which chelates and removes the mineralized inorganic component of the dentine (Fig. 5.59). Although it will flush out debris, EDTA does not dissolve organic matter, so it should be used in conjunction with NaOCl.

Placement of intracanal medicaments

Root canals are dried with paper points to remove irrigant before placing an intracanal medicament. Paper points of increased taper are useful as fewer are required to dry the root canal (Fig. 5.60). The medicament may be placed into the root canal using ISO size 10 files, but ideally a spiral filler or a proprietary medicament in syringe with fine tip is used to ensure that the root canal is completely filled.

Agitation of irrigant

Recapitulation should be carried out each time fresh irrigant is introduced during instrumentation. When instrumentation has been completed, the irrigant should be agitated by the introduction of a well-fitting GP cone into the root canal and moving the cone up and down in the root canal with 3–4 mm push-pull strokes.

Temporary restorations

A pledget of cotton wool or polytetrafluoroethylene tape should be placed in the floor of the pulp chamber and a well-adapted temporary filling should then be placed before removing the rubber dam.

Summary points

- Root canal preparation involves simultaneous mechanical and chemical preparation of the root canal system (chemomechanical debridement).

- The aims of chemomechanical debridement are to remove microbes, pulpal remnants, and organic debris from the root canal system, and create an optimal shape to allow a well-compacted root canal filling to be placed into the root canal system.

- Mechanical preparation involves several stages which should be carried out methodically. The coronal portion of the root canal should be prepared before progressing apically.

- The working length can be reliably and predictably determined using an electronic apex locator (EAL) or a working length radiograph. For optimal accuracy, it is recommended that a combination of the two methods is utilized.

- The majority of endodontic files are made of either stainless or nickel-titanium (NiTi). There are many advantages to NiTi files including greater flexibility, greater resistance to fracture, and built-in taper. They are not a panacea and should be used in conjunction with stainless steel files.

- Chemical preparation of the root canal system is primarily achieved using irrigants that are delivered into the root canal system. Sodium hypochlorite (NaOCl) meets many of the ideal properties of an irrigant: principally, it is antimicrobial and has an organic tissue dissolving capacity. EDTA may also be used to remove the smear layer. Irrigants should be agitated to increase their efficacy. Chemical preparation may also be achieved using a medicament.

Suggested further reading

Bhuva B (2011) Working length determination (Section 4. Case 4.5). In: Patel S and Duncan HF (eds) *Pitt Ford's Problem-Based Learning in Endodontology*, 1st edn, pp. 137–46. Chichester: Wiley-Blackwell.

European Society of Endodontology (2006) Quality guidelines for endodontic treatment: consensus report of the European Society of Endodontology. *International Endodontic Journal* **39**: 921–30.

Patel S (2011) Disinfection of the root canal system (Section 4. Case 4.4). In: Patel S and Duncan HF (eds) *Pitt Ford's Problem-Based Learning in Endodontology*, 1st edn, pp. 129–36 Chichester: Wiley-Blackwell.

Peters OA and Peters CI (2011) Cleaning and shaping of the root canal system. In: Hargreaves KM, Cohen S and Berman LH (eds) *Pathways of the Pulp*, 10th edn, pp. 283–348. Missouri: Mosby Elsevier.

Schafer E (2011) Instrumentation of the root canal system (Section 4. Case 4.2). In: Patel S and Duncan HF(eds) *Pitt Ford's Problem-Based Learning in Endodontology*, 1st edn, pp. 110–7. Chichester: Wiley-Blackwell.

Online Resource Centre

To help you to develop and apply your knowledge and skills further, we have provided interactive learning resources online at http://www.oxfordtextbooks.co.uk/orc/patel/

6

Root canal filling

Conor Durack
and Edward Brady

Chapter contents

Introduction

This chapter will introduce the underlying theory of root canal filling before exploring how this transfers to clinical practice. It is important that you read the whole chapter to understand how the theory and practice of root canal filling are related. Root canal filling, traditionally known as obturation, is a term used to describe the placement of an appropriate material in the chemomechanically prepared (disinfected) root canal system.

Why is it necessary to fill root canals?

The complexity of the root canal system is such that even the most advanced and contemporary preparation and irrigation techniques are unable to consistently eliminate all microbes.

The objectives of root canal filling are to:

- Entomb (completely surround with the filling material) any microbes remaining within the root canal system following preparation, thereby denying them access to the periapical tissues and any intracanal nutritional sources;

- Completely seal all anatomical portals of entry/exit to the root canal system and prevent access of nutritional sources (e.g. periapical tissue fluid, saliva) into the root canal system;

- Prevent reinfection of the root canal system by denying access to oral microbes (i.e. coronal leakage from saliva contamination) (Fig. 6.1).

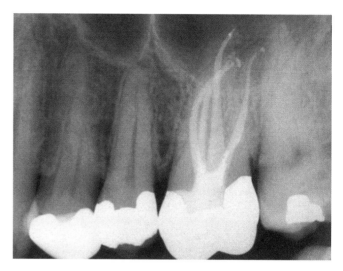

Figure 6.1 Periapical radiograph of a well compacted root canal filling in a maxillary first molar tooth. The root canal filling is homogenous, occupies the entire root canal system, and does not contain voids.

When should root canals be filled?

Background

Root canal systems should only be filled once chemomechanical preparation is complete. Theoretically, the most appropriate time to fill is when there are fewest microbes in the root canal system. Historically, infected teeth were subjected to microbiological sampling techniques to identify the presence of microbes prior to root canal filling. When the results were negative it was deemed time to fill. Unfortunately, the tests performed were time-consuming and impracticable and have now been largely abandoned.

Today, decisions on the timing of root canal filling may be influenced by pulp vitality and the microbiological status of the pulp space (based largely on preoperative radiographic information) before the root canal is accessed. Information on pulp vitality may be obtained from sensibility testing and clinical symptoms (e.g. symptoms of pulpitis), while the presence of a periapical radiolucency associated with a non-vital tooth is an indication that the root canal space is infected. The root canal system of a tooth with an irreversibly inflamed, but still vital (non-infected) pulp may be more appropriately prepared and filled at the same appointment. This will reduce the period of time the tooth is restored with a temporary restoration, thereby limiting the risk of coronal leakage. On the other hand, a tooth with an infected necrotic pulp theoretically may benefit from an interappointment antimicrobial medicament, placed in the root canals after preparation, in order to further reduce the number of microbes in the root canal system.

Despite these simplistic guidelines there are very few biological contraindications to preparing and filling the root canals in one visit and often clinician preference and opinion plays a role in the decision-making. In addition, there are other factors, which should be taken in to consideration before a definitive decision is made on when to fill the root canals (see 'Factors influencing the most appropriate time to fill', below).

Single and multiple visit root canal treatment

Single visit root canal treatment is a term used to describe the complete preparation and filling of the root canal system in one appointment. Multiple visit root canal treatment involves the preparation and filling of the root canal system over two or more appointments—generally the preparation is completed at the first appointment and the root canals are filled at the next appointment. When root canal treatment is carried out in multiple visits the root canals should be dressed with an antimicrobial medicament between appointments (interappointment medicament). Calcium hydroxide is the interappointment medicament of choice.

What are the factors influencing the most appropriate time to fill the root canal system?

The following factors should be considered before deciding on the timing of root canal filling (Table 6.1):

Status of the pulp and periapical tissues

For the reasons discussed above, it is generally accepted that a single visit treatment is appropriate for teeth with vital pulps (e.g. teeth undergoing

Table 6.1 Simple guidelines on when to fill root canals

Single visit

- Vital (uninfected) teeth, time permitting

Single or multi visit

- Infected or necrotic teeth which are not acutely symptomatic
- Teeth with large open apices
- Reasons specific to patient management

Multi visit

- Teeth in which the root canals cannot be dried
- Acutely symptomatic teeth associated with infected, necrotic root canals, and/or periapical abscess
- Procedurally difficult cases where there has been inadequate time for chemomechanical preparation

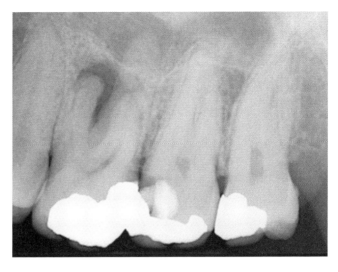

Figure 6.3 Periapical radiograph of a maxillary molar tooth with an associated periapical radiolucency. The tooth was diagnosed with chronic periapical periodontitis associated with an infected and necrotic root canal system.

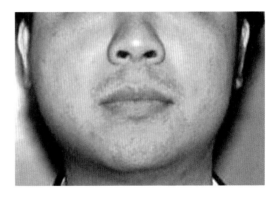

Figure 6.4 Clinical photograph of a patient with a swelling on the right side of his face caused by an acute periapical abscess.

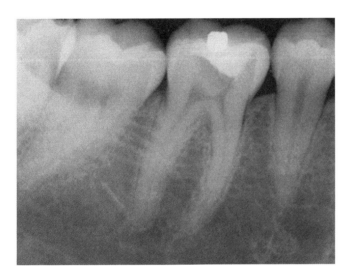

Figure 6.2 Periapical radiograph of a mandibular molar without an associated periapical radiolucency. The tooth was diagnosed with irreversible pulpitis associated with gross caries underneath an existing restoration and was treated in a single visit.

elective root canal treatment, teeth with irreversible pulpitis, etc.), time and patient/procedural factors permitting (Fig. 6.2).

Root canal systems which are infected, (i.e. teeth showing radiographic signs of periapical periodontitis) are more challenging to disinfect (Fig. 6.3). This is particularly true in teeth which require revision of failing root canal treatments as they tend to be infected with very persistent microbes, which are especially difficult to eradicate. Scientific evidence has shown that an interappointment calcium hydroxide medicament significantly reduces the microbial load of the root canal system when compared to root canal preparation and irrigation with sodium hypochlorite (NaOCl) alone. Logically one might therefore expect better success rates for multiple visit root canal treatment. However, research has, so far, failed to show any difference in the outcome of root canal treatment whether it is carried out in a single visit or in multiple visits using calcium hydroxide as an interappointment medicament.

Therefore, a decision on the most appropriate time to fill, *based on the status of the pulp and periapical tissues alone*, is ultimately at the discretion of the clinician.

Patient's signs and symptoms

When a patient presents for treatment with acute symptoms, such as pain and swelling associated with pulp necrosis and acute periapical abscess (Fig. 6.4), it may be prudent to prepare the root canals at the first visit and fill the root canals at a subsequent appointment when the patient's symptoms have resolved. This is to allow easier management of these patients should the symptoms persist or worsen following the initial visit.

Flare-up

A flare-up can be defined as a post-operative episode of pain and/or swelling following root canal treatment, severe enough to require unscheduled dental treatment to manage the symptoms. There is conflicting scientific evidence relating to the occurrence of flare-ups when root canal treatment is carried out in single or multiple visits. Some research reports a higher incidence of flare-ups with single visit treatment while other research suggests a higher incidence with multiple visit treatment. What is clear, however, is that post-operative pain and/or swelling is more likely to occur when the patient presents with preoperative acute symptoms. In such cases it may be more prudent to carry out root canal treatment over more than one visit.

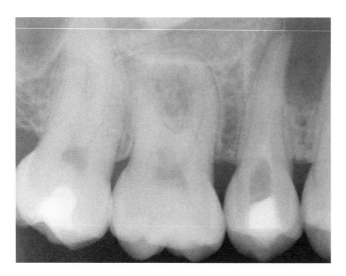

Figure 6.5 Periapical radiograph of a maxillary first molar tooth with a complex root morphology.

Procedural difficulty

Some teeth may be more difficult to treat than others and the complexity of the case may result in the need for multiple visits due to time constraints. Examples of cases which may be more time-consuming include those involving teeth with difficult anatomy (Fig. 6.5), cases in which there is difficulty achieving effective anaesthesia, and retreatment cases in which the existing root canal filling material is challenging to remove (Fig. 6.6).

On occasion, following root canal preparation, blood or inflammatory exudate may continue to seep into the root canal system ('weeping' root canals) such that the root canal system cannot be adequately dried. In these situations root canal filling should be deferred and the root canals should be dressed with calcium hydroxide until such time as they can be made completely dry. Incorporating blood or inflammatory exudate into the root canal filling compromises the seal and provides microbes with nutrient sources and space to multiply.

Filling root canals of teeth with open apices can be challenging as the natural resistance (i.e. root canal taper) to compaction of the root canal filling is no longer present (Fig. 6.7). The traditional method for creating an apical barrier in these cases ('apexification') involves long-term medicament of the root canal system with calcium hydroxide, in order to stimulate calcific barrier formation at the root-end prior to root canal filling. This is carried out over multiple visits, is time-consuming, potentially weakens the tooth, and has been largely superseded by apexification using calcium silicate cements (see section 'Filling root canals with open apices'). Apexification with calcium silicate cements is advantageous in that it can be carried out in single or multiple visits and the procedure itself does not further weaken the tooth.

Patient management

Patient preference, circumstances, and/or medical conditions may have a bearing on the timing of root canal filling. For example, a patient with severe haemophilia may require clotting factor cover prior to the administration of an inferior alveolar nerve block. This may be expensive and difficult to coordinate with the treating haematology department. It

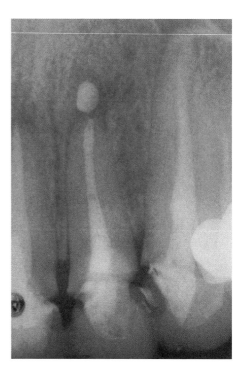

Figure 6.6 Periapical radiograph of symptomatic maxillary central incisor, lateral incisor, and canine teeth which have been filled with a hard setting paste which proved challenging and time-consuming to subsequently remove.

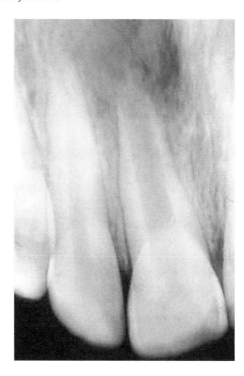

Figure 6.7 Periapical radiograph of a maxillary central incisor with incomplete root development and an associated periapical radiolucency.

would be pragmatic in these circumstances to carry out root canal treatment of a mandibular molar in a single visit, if at all possible.

Some patients may find it difficult to attend for multiple appointments due to work/personal commitments and may request that the treatment

Table 6.2 Examples of root canal sealers

Sealer base-material	Properties	Examples
Zinc oxide-eugenol	• Currently the most widely used type of sealer • Successfully used over many years • Demonstrates antimicriobial properties	Tubliseal (Kerr, Romulus, MI, USA) Pulp Canal Sealer (Kerr, Romulus, MI, USA)
Calcium hydroxide	• Designed to release calcium hydroxide over long periods in order to provide antimicrobial and osteogenic (bone-forming) benefits, but these have not been demonstrated • The sealer needs to be soluble in order to release calcium hydroxide, which may result in the formation of voids in the root canal filling • Poor cohesive strength	Apexit (Ivoclar Vivadent AG, Schaan, Liechtenstein Sealapex (Kerr, Romulus, MI, USA)
Resin	• Long working times • Adheres well to dentine initially but contracts away from the root canal wall on setting • Flows well • Easy to remove	AH Plus (Dentsply Maillefer, Ballaigues, Switzerland)

is carried out in one visit. Patients with back complaints may prefer multiple shorter appointments rather than a single prolonged appointment in order to avoid the discomfort of lying in a dental chair for extended periods.

Reasons specific to patient management may therefore dictate whether a tooth is treated in single or multiple visits. Exceptions to this are cases in which the root canals cannot be dried following preparation and cases where acute symptoms are caused by necrotic, infected pulps or periapical abscess. In these cases treatment should be carried out in multiple visits regardless of patient circumstances.

What materials are used for root canal filling?

There are various endodontic materials available for filling root canals. Regardless of the specific materials used a root canal filling should consist of a core material and a sealer.

Root canal sealers

The main function of a root canal sealer is to fill the space between the core filling material and the root canal wall. Sealers also fill accessory and lateral root canals and the space between individual root canal filling points when cold lateral compaction is used. Root canal sealers can be classified according to their base material (Table 6.2). Several groups of sealers exist, these include: zinc oxide eugenol-based sealers, e.g. Pulp Canal Sealer (Kerr, Romulus, MI, USA) and Kerr Tubliseal (Kerr) (Fig. 6.8); calcium hydroxide-based sealers, e.g. Sealapex (Kerr); Apexit (Ivoclar Vivadent AG, Schaan, Liechtenstein) (Fig. 6.9); and resin-based sealers, e.g. AH Plus (Dentsply-Maillefer, Ballaigues, Switzerland) (Fig. 6.10). Glass ionomer-based sealers, e.g. Ketac-Endo (3M ESPE, St. Paul, MN, USA) and silicone-based sealers, e.g. RoekoSeal (Roeko/Coltènè/Whaledent, Langenau, Germany) are also available but are not commonly used.

An ideal root canal sealer will:

• be biocompatible;
• be non-toxic and non-mutagenic;
• be safe to use;
• be inexpensive;
• have a long shelf-life;
• be easy to handle and have an adequate working time;
• be bactericidal or at least bacteriostatic;
• be radiopaque;
• be dimensionally stable on setting;
• be insoluble in tissue fluids;
• not stain the tooth;
• be easily removed should root canal treatment need to be revised.

No sealer currently available demonstrates all of these properties. All sealers are slightly toxic to the periapical tissues when initially mixed but the toxicity reduces greatly when they are set. All sealers are resorbed by tissue fluids to varying degrees. Healing of the periapical tissues may be delayed (but not prevented) in the presence of extruded root canal sealer.

Root canal core filling materials

At present gutta-percha (GP) is the most suitable core material to predictably and simply fill the root canal system. The ideal root canal filling material should:

• be biocompatible;
• be non-toxic and non-mutagenic;

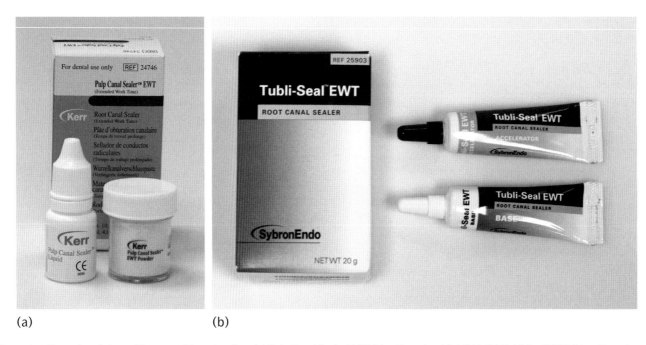

Figure 6.8 Examples of zinc-oxide eugenol-based sealers: (a) Pulp Canal Sealer EWT (Kerr Romulus, MI, USA); (b) Tubli-Seal EWT (Kerr, Romulus, MI, USA).

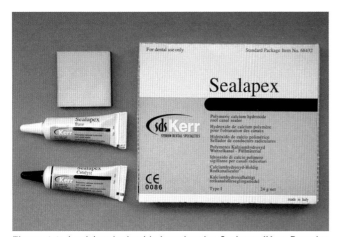

Figure 6.9 A calcium hydroxide-based sealer, Sealapex (Kerr, Romulus, MI, USA).

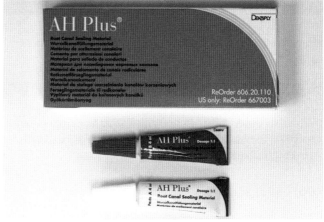

Figure 6.10 A resin-based sealer, AH Plus (Dentsply-Maillefer, Ballaigues, Switzerland).

- be safe to use;
- be inexpensive;
- have a long shelf-life;
- be easy to handle and have a long working time;
- be bactericidal or at least bacteriostatic;
- be sterile;
- be easy to introduce into the root canal;
- conform and adapt to the irregular shape of the root canals;
- be radiopaque;
- be dimensionally stable on setting;
- be insoluble in tissue fluids;
- not stain the tooth;
- be easily removed should root canal treatment need to be revised.

No currently available core material demonstrates all these properties. All core materials leak to some extent and it is essential that the root canals are properly cleaned and shaped prior to root canal filling. Inadequately cleaned and shaped root canals are difficult to fill properly.

Gutta-percha

The most commonly used root canal filling material is gutta-percha (GP). It remains the root canal filling material of choice, as it has many of the properties of an ideal root canal filling material. Gutta-percha is a polymer derived from the taban tree and is an isomer of rubber. It is modified for use in endodontics; the final root canal filling material

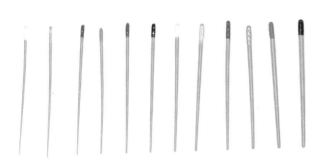

Figure 6.11 International Organization of Standardization (ISO) standard sized GP points with a uniform taper of 0.02, sizes 15–80 (left to right).

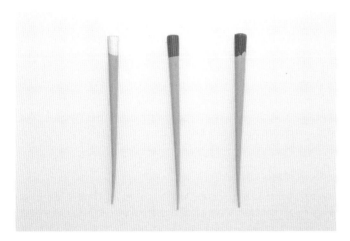

Figure 6.12 Greater taper GP points, ProTaper (Dentsply-Maillefer, Ballaigues, Switzerland). The F1 ProTaper GP point (yellow head, and left of picture) has a tip diameter equivalent to that of an ISO size 20 GP point but has a taper of 0.07. The F2 ProTaper GP point (red head, and middle of picture) has a tip diameter equivalent to that of an ISO size 25 GP point, but has a taper of 0.08. The F3 ProTaper GP point (blue head, and right of picture) has a tip diameter equivalent to that of an ISO size 30 GP point, but has a taper of 0.09.

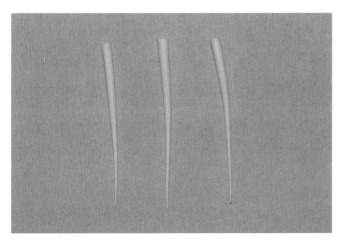

Figure 6.13 Polymer-based points (Propoint; Smartseal DRFP, Stamford, UK).

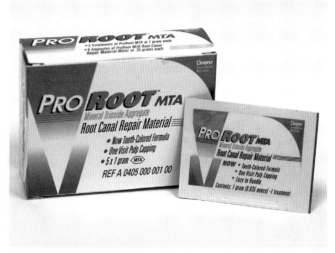

(a)

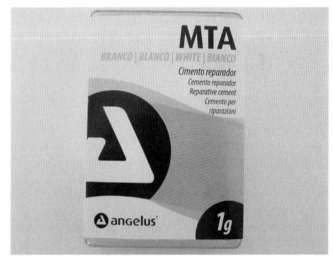

(b)

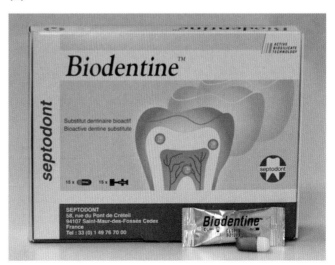

(c)

Figure 6.14 Calcium silicate cements: (a) ProRoot MTA (Dentsply Tulsa Dental, Tulsa, OK, USA); (b) MTA-Angelus (Angelus, Londrina-PR, Brazil) (c) Biodentine (Septodont, Saint-Maur-des-Fossés, France) calcium silicate cement.

is composed of zinc oxide (60–75 per cent), unrefined GP (19–22 per cent), opacifiers (barium sulphate (1–17 per cent)), and waxes and resins (1–4 per cent). Gutta-percha can be used at room temperature, with heat or with softening agents (e.g. chloroform). It is used in conjunction with a sealer to produce a homogenous dense mass to seal the root canal space. Gutta-percha is manufactured in International Organization of Standardization (ISO) standard sizes with a uniform taper of 0.02 (Fig. 6.11), and various non-standard sizes and tapers (Fig. 6.12).

Polymer-based materials

Polymer-based materials have been introduced as alternative root canal filling materials in the past number of years. These use a thermoplastic synthetic polymer (Fig. 6.13), which contains bioactive glass and radiopaque fillers, as the core material. They are used in conjunction with resin-based sealer systems. Polymer-based materials have similar handling properties to GP and can be placed in root canals using similar techniques. The intended benefits of the polymer-based systems are improved sealing of the root canal system. When the root canal walls are conditioned with a self-etch primer, a resin-based sealer is introduced into the root canals and the polymer-based core is then inserted. The sealer is mechanically retained to the etched root canal walls and also bonds to the core, theoretically producing a homogenous 'monoblock'. The ability of polymer-based materials to perform as well as GP over long periods has not been established.

Calcium silicate cements

Calcium silicate cements are a group of contemporary endodontic filling materials which include Mineral Trioxide Aggregate (MTA) and Biodentine (Septodont, Saint-Maur-des-Fossés, France) (Fig. 6.14). Their potential uses in endodontics are diverse. MTA was the first calcium silicate cement developed for use in endodontics. It was initially developed as a root-end filling material, but due to its biocompatibility and its ability to set in the presence of moisture it has become the first choice material used for apexification procedures on teeth with open apices. Following the creation of an apical barrier of MTA the material can then be used to fill the remainder of the root canal, if desired. MTA is the only dental material which is known to promote the deposition of cementum immediately adjacent to it when it is exposed to the periradicular tissues. It has been the subject of intense research since the 1990s and has been used widely in clinical endodontic practice for more than a decade with unparalleled success. However, MTA does have some disadvantages. These include its consistency, which makes handling relatively difficult, and its propensity to cause a grey discolouration of the crown of tooth when it is used as a root canal filling material, apexification material or pulp capping material. MTA was originally developed as a grey powder. Attempts to overcome the issues of discolouration have seen the development of a white MTA powder in recent years. MTA is manufactured under two main brand names: Pro-Root MTA (Dentsply Tulsa Dental, Tulsa, OK, USA) and MTA-Angelus (Angelus, Londrina-PR, Brazil).

Biodentine (Septodont, Saint-Maur-des-Fossés, France) is a newer calcium silicate cement, which has been developed as a dental material. Its potential uses in endodontics are similar to those of MTA. It also has an improved setting time and handling properties which some clinicians may find more favourable than those of MTA. It is a promising material; however, research on its use in endodontics is relatively sparse. In addition, its radiodensity is a concern as it is not always easily identifiable on radiographs.

Historical materials

Silver points (Fig. 6.15) were popular during a period when it was generally accepted that root canal treatment was very difficult to carry out. Silver points were easily introduced into the root canals and were stiff enough to reach the working length, but did not result in complete

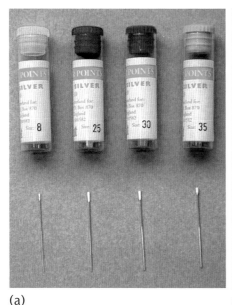

(a)

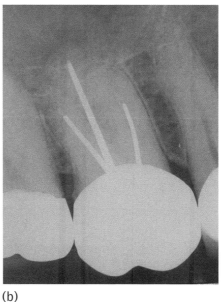

(b)

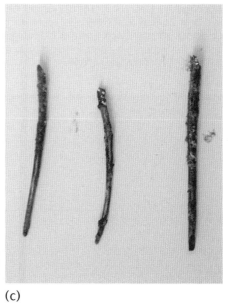

(c)

Figure 6.15 Silver points: (a) packaged silver points with varying tip sizes; (b) periapical radiograph of a maxillary molar tooth with an associated periapical radiolucency. The root canals have been filled with silver points. (c) Silver points retrieved from root canals. They have corroded and are a darker colour.

filling of the root canal space. Due to their rigidity and ease of placement, adequate preparation and shaping of the root canals was often neglected. In addition, silver points corrode in contact with saliva and tissue fluids, resulting in the production of potentially cytotoxic breakdown products. As a consequence, treatment failures associated with silver point root canal fillings were common.

Acrylic points were historically used in a manner similar to silver points, but they displayed many of the disadvantages of their silver counterparts.

Pastes, including formaldehyde pastes (e.g. N2, Endomethasone, SPAD), were also once used to fill root canals. Due to their toxicity and unpredictable flow properties they are no longer used.

What is the apical extent of an ideal root canal filling?

The root canal filling should extend through the full length of the root canal, from the root canal entrance to the apical constriction (Fig. 6.16). This will help prevent reinfection of the root canal system by microbes. The apical constriction can be up to 2.5 mm coronal to the radiographic apex of the tooth so a root canal filling which appears flush with the apex on a radiograph may actually have extruded through the apical constriction. It is therefore important to use an electronic apex locator (EAL), tactile feedback, and, if necessary, working length radiographs to accurately gauge the position of the apical constriction. A master cone radiograph is also essential prior to filling the root canals.

There are several root canal filling techniques currently in vogue and they all aim to produce a dense, homogenously filled root canal system without voids. The use of cold compaction techniques should ensure control, in particular, of the length of the root canal filling. The root canal filling material should reach a predetermined length and be well adapted to the root canal walls.

Selection of the master point is a crucial step in root canal filling. The master point should fit snugly at the appropriate position in the apical portion of the root canal. The term 'tug-back' has been used to describe the snug fit and slight resistance to withdrawal that the master cone should exhibit when tried in and removed. It is assumed that this tug-back is always at the full working length but it may in fact be at a more coronal point in the root canal, due to the complexities of the root canal system and curvatures in planes not shown on the radiographs.

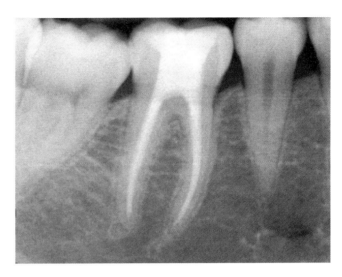

Figure 6.16 Periapical radiograph of a mandibular first molar tooth with a well extended and compacted root canal filing. Note that the root canal filling in the distal root terminates approximately 1.5 mm from the radiographic apex. This is the position of the apical constriction in that root canal, as determined using an electronic apex locator (EAL). The apical constriction in the mesial root canals is approximately 0.5 mm from the radiographic apex of the mesial root.

Care should be taken to avoid the use of small GP points, which may inadvertently extend beyond the working length and, if forced into the periapical tissues, may induce an inflammatory or foreign body reaction.

Foundations of clinical practice

The remainder of this chapter provides criteria for successful root canal filling using the most common techniques. It should be remembered that the quality of the root canal filling can only be as good as the preparation will allow.

Which size gutta-percha point should be used?

The International Organization for Standardization (ISO) first established international standards for endodontic instruments in 1974. Traditional stainless steel files used today (e.g. K-Flexofile, K-Flex, Hedström) are manufactured to a tip size and taper standardized by the ISO (see Chapter 5).

Many nickel-titanium (NiTi) hand and machine-driven (rotary and reciprocating) files are manufactured with varying tapers (depending on the manufacturer and specific instrument type), which do not conform to the ISO specifications. However, most manufacturers will produce GP points, paper points and finger spreaders to match the corresponding sizes and tapers of these files.

In simple terms, when filling a root canal, the master GP point should be matched to the size of the master apical file. If root canal preparation has been carried out with files that have an increased or varying taper (i.e. with NiTi files), a master GP point that matches the apical size and taper of the preparation should be chosen as a starting point. An ISO standard sized GP point should be used if the root canal is to be filled using lateral compaction.

Root canal sealer placement

There are a variety of methods of root canal sealer placement. These include sealer application with paper points, the master GP point, hand files, ultrasonic files, or spiral fillers. The following are basic steps in sealer placement using the various techniques:

- When using paper points or the master GP point as the sealer carrier, the apical 5–6 mm of the point is evenly and lightly coated with sealer. The point is then introduced into the root canal to the working length and moved very gently up and down (1–2 mm) with additional lateral movement against the root canal walls. Where the paper point is used as the carrier, this is then removed and the master GP point is placed to the full working length. Where the master GP point itself is used as the carrier, it is fully seated to the working length after sealer placement.

Lateral compaction

The technique described here is widely taught and understood. It is simple, predictable, and can be performed with the minimum of gadgetry. Lateral compaction is still the reference standard to which other root canal filling techniques are compared. Many of the newer techniques of root canal filling that have been developed (and may come to attract you!) are often dependent on expensive pieces of equipment and the acquisition

While GP is the most commonly used core root canal filling material, polymer-based materials are also available and may be employed to fill root canals using any of the techniques which are suitable for the compaction of GP.

- When a file is used as the sealer carrier, it is important to choose a sterile file with a tip diameter which can be accommodated at the full working length—the master apical file or a size smaller will generally suffice. The apical 5–6 mm of the file is coated in the sealer, as before. The file is inserted into the root canal to the full working length and rotated anticlockwise with additional circumferential movement. The file is then withdrawn as it is continually rotated.

- Alternatively, spiral fillers or ultrasonically activated files may be used to apply the sealer to the root canal. There is an inherent risk of instrument fracture when these techniques are used inappropriately, and they are rarely used for this purpose.

of particular skills. They do not necessarily produce better clinical results, though they may be quicker and, in experienced hands, less tiring to use. The principal of lateral compaction is that lateral pressure applied with a spreader to a GP point will compact the point and create space for the placement of accessory GP points. The process is repeated until the root canal filling is well compacted and fills the entire root canal.

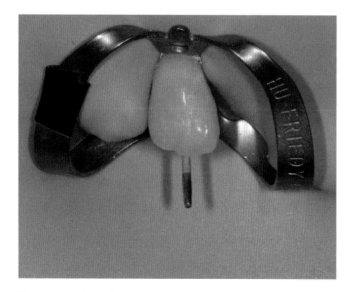

Figure 6.17 Master GP point seated in the root canal, prior to filling using cold lateral compaction.

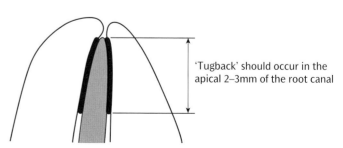

'Tugback' should occur in the apical 2–3mm of the root canal

Figure 6.18 Diagram illustrating the concept of 'tugback'.

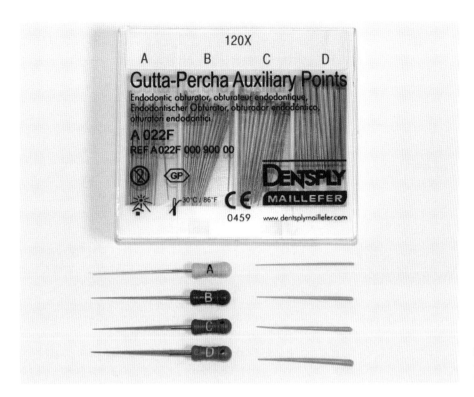

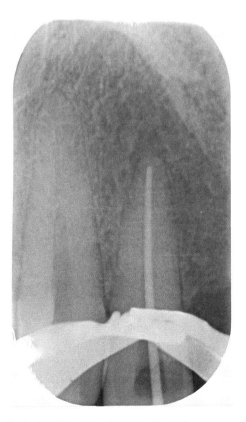

Figure 6.19 Finger spreaders and matching GP points (Dentsply-Maillefer, Ballaigues, Switzerland).

The criteria for successful root canal filling using lateral compaction are:

- A master GP point is chosen that corresponds to the size of the master apical file. Try this in a wet root canal (this provides lubrication), using locking tweezers (Fig. 6.17). Feel for 'tug-back'. Effective tug-back is the resistance felt when the GP point binds in the apical region of the root canal (Fig. 6.18). ISO standard sized GP points should be used for cold lateral compaction.

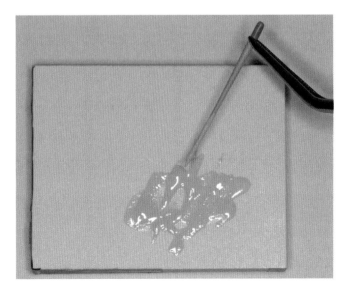

Figure 6.21 Root canal sealer applied evenly to the apical third of the master GP point.

Figure 6.20 Master GP point periapical radiograph.

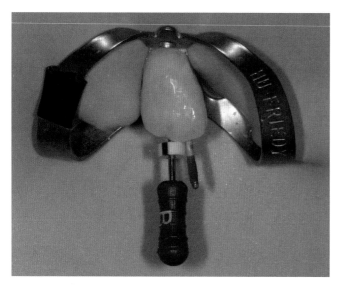

Figure 6.22 The appropriate sized finger spreader is inserted into the root canal beside the master GP point and extends to within 1 mm of the apical extent of the master GP point.

- A finger spreader is selected that fits comfortably to within 1 mm of the working length. Finger spreaders come in various sizes depending on the brand selected (Fig. 6.19). Use a silicone stop to gauge its length, then remove the spreader and confirm its length.
- A master point radiograph should be taken to confirm the length of the master GP point (Fig. 6.20).
- A successful master point should bind within 1 mm of the full working length with tug-back—it is assumed that the pressure of lateral compaction will allow up to 1 mm of further apical movement.
- Dry the root canal with paper points.

- Mix the sealer and apply it to the root canal wall (see the section on sealer placement). Apply more sealer to the apical third of the GP point (Fig. 6.21) and introduce it gently but firmly to the working length.
- Insert the finger spreader alongside the GP point (Fig. 6.22). If the root canal is curved, the finger spreader should be inserted along the outermost side of the root canal—this is less likely to result in the sharp tip of the finger spreader engaging the GP point and leading to the inadvertent removal of the point when the finger spreader is withdrawn (Fig. 6.23). Maintaining firm apical pressure on the finger spreader for 15 seconds will laterally and apically compact the GP.
- Rotate the finger spreader clockwise and anticlockwise through 40° (or so), for several seconds whilst maintaining apical pressure before removing it.
- Insert a corresponding sized accessory GP point in the space created by the finger spreader. This accessory point should have a small amount of sealer on its apical 3–4 mm prior to insertion.
- Remove residual sealer from the finger spreader and insert it again into the root canal as before followed by an accessory GP point (Fig. 6.24) until the root canal is fully filled (Fig. 6.25).
- A mid-fill radiograph may also be of use to assess the filling before the root canal is completely filled (Fig. 6.26). In this way necessary adjustments can be made to the filling prior to completion of the task.
- Take a post-fill radiograph (Fig. 6.27). This should show a dense, uniformly radiopaque mass within the root canal system, terminating at the apical extent of the preparation. There should be no obvious voids in the apical- and mid-thirds of the root canal filling.
- Sear off the excess GP at the base of the pulp chamber with a heated instrument and compact the coronal GP mass to below the level of the cemento–enamel junction (Fig. 6.27) using an endodontic plugger (Fig. 6.28).

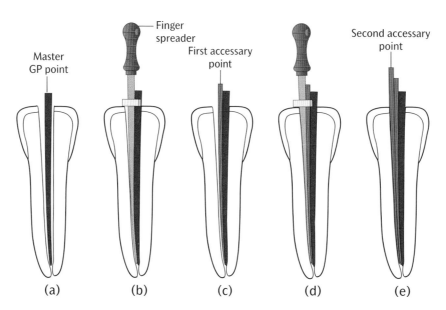

(a)   (b)   (c)   (d)   (e)

Figure 6.23 Cold lateral compaction. (a) Master GP point lightly coated with sealer and seated into the root canal; (b) finger spreader inserted between outer aspect of curved root canal and master GP point; (c) accessory GP point seated into space created by finger spreader; (d and e) stages (b) and (c) are repeated until the finger spreader cannot create any more space in the mid-portion of the root canal for insertion of accessory GP points.

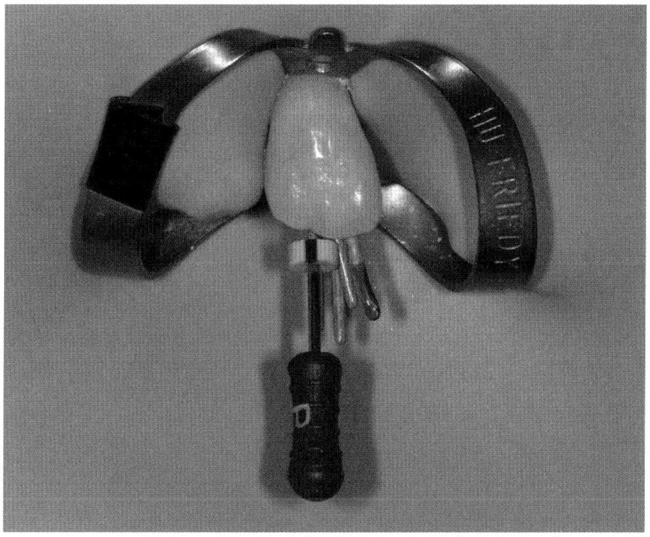

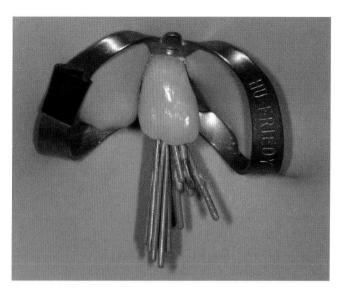

Figure 6.24 The finger spreader is seated in the root canal with the master GP point and accessory points. The finger spreader compacts the GP in the root canal to create space for accessory points.

Figure 6.25 The root canal has been filled with GP points and cannot accommodate any more.

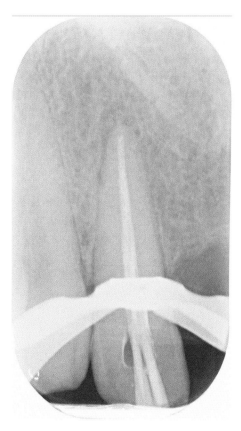

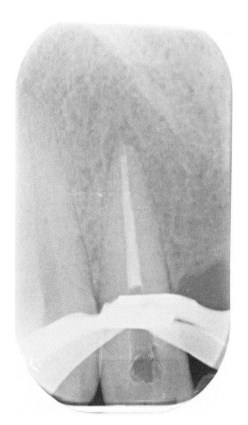

Figure 6.26 A periapical radiograph taken approximately halfway through the process of cold lateral compaction. Radiographic assessment at this stage gives the clinician an indication as to how well the root canal filling is compacted. Alterations can then be made to the filling as necessary.

Figure 6.27 A periapical radiograph taken at the completion of root canal filling. The purpose of the radiograph is to assess the quality of the filling, prior to the provision of the core. This particular post-fill radiograph was taken after searing off the excess GP and then compacting the GP in the root canal. The radiograph can be taken prior to this. Note the level of the coronal extent of the filling, below the cemento–enamel junction.

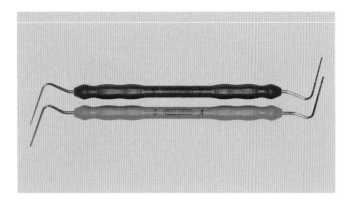

Figure 6.28 Machtou endodontic pluggers (Dentsply-Mailleger, Ballaigues, Switzerland): sizes 1 and 2 (red handle) and sizes 3 and 4 (grey handle).

- Where two root canals fuse, the root canal which has been prepared to the full working length should be filled first, after which the second root canal may be filled.

- Seal the entrances to the root canals with IRM (Dentsply Caulk, Milford, DE, USA). The antimicrobial nature of this material will help to prevent penetration of microbes into the filled root canals, should the integrity of the coronal restoration be breached. Place a base of glass ionomer on the floor of the pulp chamber.

- Ideally, an immediate core restoration should be placed and a post-operative radiograph should be taken (Fig. 6.29).

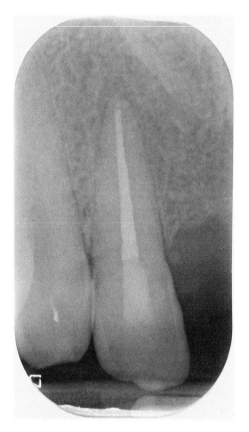

Figure 6.29 Post-operative periapical radiograph.

Creation of a customized master gutta-percha point

Customized GP points are created when the dimensions of the master GP point do not match the dimensions of the prepared root canal apically. This occurs in situations such as when the root apex has undergone resorption, or in situations where the apical portion of the root canal is irregular in shape.

A customized master GP point adapted to fit the exact dimensions of the apical portion of the root canal can be created as follows for teeth with larger or open apices (Fig. 6.30):

- A master GP point, which binds in the root canal 1–2 mm short of the working length is chosen;

- The apical 3 mm of the GP point is softened in a solvent, such as chloroform;

- The softened GP point is introduced into the root canal and manipulated apically until the working length is reached;

- The softened GP point is left *in situ* until it hardens and is then removed from the root canal with a locking tweezers. A note must be made of the exact orientation of the GP point in the root canal before it is removed, as once the sealer is applied, the GP point must go back into the root canal in the same position, so that it fits the root canal exactly. To this end, the point must not be released from the locking tweezers until the sealer has been applied and the point has been fitted.

Wider root canals may require the chair-side fabrication of a large master cone before it is customized as outlined above. This is achieved by heating several GP points and rolling them into a large single cone using a spatula and a glass slab.

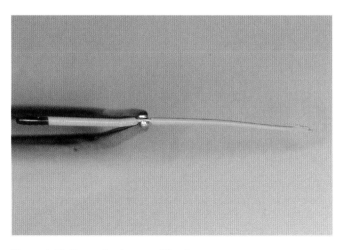

Figure 6.30 Customized master GP point.

Thermoplastic compaction

Heat can be used when filling the root canal system to produce a more homogenous and dense root canal filling. There are a variety of techniques, which involve the use of heat and these are collectively referred to as 'thermoplastic compaction'. These techniques rely on either warming the GP prior to inserting it into the prepared root canal (carrier-based systems), or warming the GP once it has been inserted into the root canal (e.g. warm vertical compaction). Table 6.3 summarizes the advantages and disadvantages of warm and cold root canal filling techniques.

Warm lateral compaction

Essentially the steps involved are the same as for cold lateral compaction, but instead of using an unheated finger spreader to compact the GP, a heated equivalent is employed. In its simplest form a finger spreader is heated using an electrical induction heater and introduced into the root canal and manipulated as for cold lateral compaction. Once compaction of the point is complete, the finger spreader will have cooled and it can be removed. Early removal of a still warm finger

Table 6.3 Summary of the advantages and disadvantages of the various root canal filling techniques

Technique	Advantages	Disadvantages
Cold lateral compaction	• The gold standard • Unparalleled by other techniques in terms of long-term success • Allows good control of the length of the filling • The filling can be revised easily if necessary • Inexpensive • Easy to master	• Time-consuming • Does not produce a homogenous mass of gutta-percha (GP) • In large root canals numerous accessory points can impair vision and accurate location of the finger spreader and subsequent points • Wedging forces produced by overzealous finger spreading insertion can lead to vertical root fractures
Warm lateral compaction	• Allows good control of length • The application of heat provides a more homogenous mass of GP • The filling can be revised easily if necessary	• Time-consuming method • In large root canals numerous accessory points can impair vision and accurate location of the finger spreader and subsequent points • Wedging forces produced by overzealous finger spreading insertion can lead to vertical root fractures
Warm vertical compaction	• Produces a homogenous mass of GP • Fills lateral and accessory anatomy • Quick method • The filling can be revised easily if necessary	• The initial cost of the equipment is expensive • The length of the root canal filling cannot be controlled as well as with cold lateral compaction • Sealer extrusion is a common occurrence
Carrier-based systems	• Fills lateral and accessory anatomy • Quick method	• The initial cost of the equipment is expensive • The length of the root canal filling cannot be controlled as well as with cold lateral compaction • Sealer extrusion is a common occurrence • Failure to heat the GP adequately may result in the obturator not seating fully • Under-prepared root canals or the incorrect angle of insertion can strip the GP from the carrier resulting in a poorly sealed canal • The filling cannot be revised without removing the carrier and GP and starting again • Removal of the carrier for revision or retreatment can be difficult • Post-preparation is more complicated than for non-carrier-based systems

spreader may result in removal of the root canal filling material. An accessory point is then placed and the procedure is repeated until the root canal is filled.

A contemporary variation involves the use of specifically designed tips, which come in a variety of sizes and can be electronically heated on command, e.g. Endotec II condenser (Medidenta, Woodside, NY, USA).

Spreaders designed for use with ultrasonic handpieces are available and can be used as an alternative to heated spreaders in warm lateral compaction of GP. The spreaders are inserted into the root canal beside the GP points and are activated without water. The activated spreaders heat up and compact the GP.

Warm vertical compaction—multiple wave technique

The aim of the warm vertical compaction technique is to produce a homogenous mass of GP, which has the potential to flow into and occupy the accessory anatomy of the root canal system. Schilder's original technique involved a repeated series of heating and compaction of GP (multiple wave compaction). Advances in technology

have seen this technique superseded by the 'continuous wave technique'.

Warm vertical compaction—continuous wave technique

Electrically heated pluggers with varying tapers designed to match the tapers of the prepared root canal were introduced by Steve Buchanan. This was called System B (SybronEndo, Orange, CA, USA) (Fig. 6.31) after the creator of the product. The pluggers heat instantly from the tip when activated and cool immediately when deactivated. A thermostat controls the temperature. The system was designed to reduce the number of stages involved in the multiple wave technique. The criteria for successful root canal filling using the continuous wave technique of warm vertical compaction are:

- The root canal is prepared and a master GP point is chosen (Fig. 6.32).
- A System B plugger is selected which extends into the root canal and binds against the walls approximately 5 mm from the working length. A silicone stop is used to mark this length on the plugger. The pluggers are malleable and will bend to the curvature of the root canal.

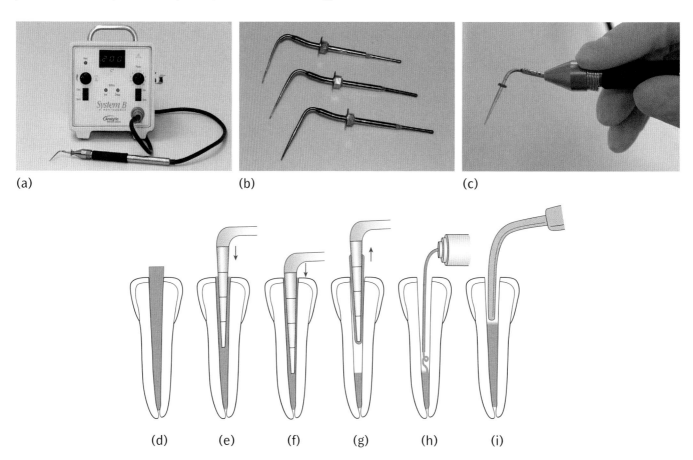

Figure 6.31 (a) System B heat source and handpiece (SybronEndo, Orange, CA, USA); (b) System B pluggers are available in several sizes; (c) the plugger is activated by pressing (and deactivated by releasing) the coil on the handpiece; (d) master GP point is inserted into the root canal; (e) an appropriate size plugger is activated and pushed apically to its predetermined length; (f) once at the predetermined length, the plugger is deactivated and firmly held against the apical GP to compensate for any shrinkage that may occur while the GP cools; (g) the plugger is activated to separate it (and remove the coronal GP) from the apical plug of GP. The remaining apical GP is then compacted with an endodontic plugger; (h) the mid- to coronal-portion of the root canal is filled with GP from a thermoplastic GP gun or extruder; (i) the coronal GP is compacted with an endodontic plugger.

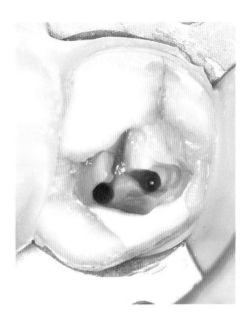

Figure 6.32 Prepared buccal root canals in a maxillary second molar, which are to be filled with GP using the continuous wave technique of warm vertical compaction.

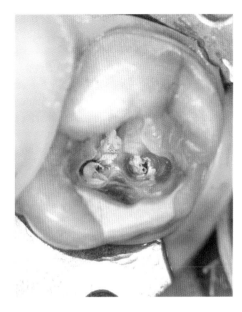

Figure 6.34 The master GP points have been seared off at the entrance to the root canals and the excess coronal GP has been removed.

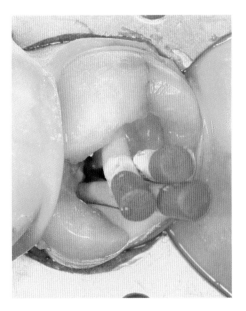

Figure 6.33 Tapered master GP points matching the taper and apical size of the prepared root canals have been chosen and are seated 0.5–1.0 mm from the working length.

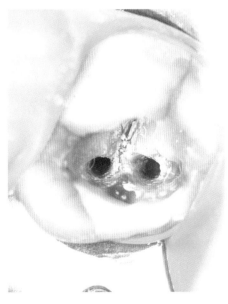

Figure 6.35 Completion of the 'downpack'. The coronal portions of the root canals are empty. The apical portions of the root canals are filled with GP, which cannot be seen in the photograph.

- Sealer is placed in the root canal and the master GP point is seated 0.5–1.0 mm from the working length (Fig. 6.33). The GP point is seared off at the entrances to the root canal using the heated plugger (Fig. 6.34).

- The power dial on the unit is set to its maximum. The plugger temperature is set to 200°C (Fig. 6.31) and is activated before being introduced into the root canal and plunged to within 2–3 mm of the binding point with firm digital pressure and in one fluid movement lasting two seconds.

- Once this depth has been reached the plugger is deactivated and firm apical pressure is maintained for 10 seconds until the GP has cooled.

- The plugger is now activated again for one second and is immediately removed from the root canal in one swift movement. The short burst of heat applied in this activation releases the plugger tip from the cooled apical plug of GP. This apical plug of GP remains in the root canal and fills the apical portion of the root canal (Fig. 6.35). The GP coronal to the plugger tip will be attached to the instrument and removed in this motion (Fig. 6.36).

- The apical plug of GP is now compacted with an endodontic plugger (Fig. 6.28). The process of filling the apical portion of the root canal in this manner is termed 'downpack'. The term is also used as a noun to describe the apical portion of GP created using this technique.

- The 'backfill' (filling of the remainder of the root canal, coronal to the downpack) is carried out using either the injection of thermoplasticized GP or incremental heating and packing of segments of GP.

- When the injection of thermoplasticized GP is chosen several products are available to carry out this function (Figs. 6.37–6.39).

- The chosen thermoplastic GP gun or extruder is activated and set to heat pellets or cartridges of GP to 200˚C.

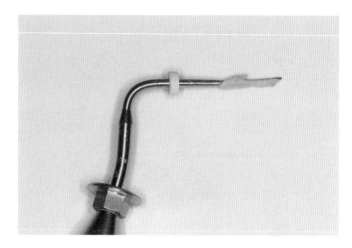

Figure 6.36 The portion of the master GP point which was occupying the coronal portion of the root canal prior to the insertion of the endodontic plugger has been removed, attached to the plugger.

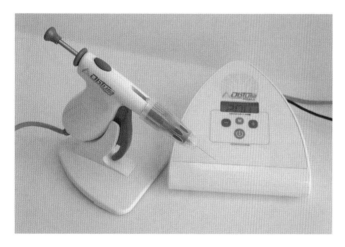

Figure 6.37 Obtura III Max system (SybronEndo, Orange, CA, USA).

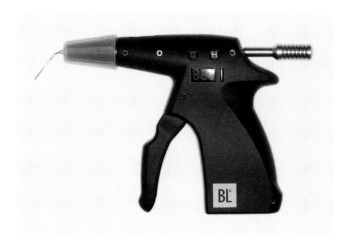

Figure 6.38 HotShot device (SybronEndo, Orange, CA, USA).

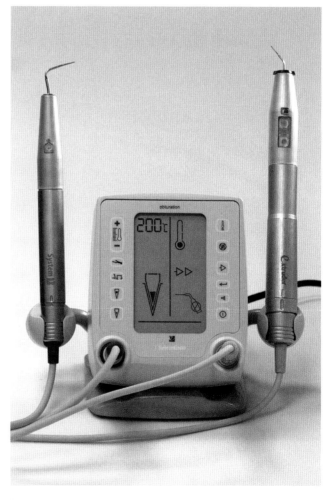

Figure 6.39 Elements obturation unit (SybronEndo, Orange, CA, USA). This comprises a System B device on the left of the main body of the unit and a thermoplasticized GP 'Extruder' on the right.

- The heated needle of the chosen thermoplastic GP gun or extruder is inserted into the root canal and sunk into the apical portion of GP (or the 'downpack'). It is held there for 5 seconds to soften the downpack and heat the inside of the root canal.

- The plasticized GP in the gun or extruder is injected by depressing a handle or button (depending on the product being used). Injection of the plasticized GP must be continued until the needle is either pushed back out of the root canal by the retreating GP or until the GP begins to flow out of the entrance to the root canal around the needle. In the latter event, the needle is withdrawn from the root canal while continuing to inject the plasticized GP.

- The plasticized GP is then compacted using an endodontic plugger (Fig. 6.28) to below the level of the cemento–enamel junction (Fig. 6.40).

- The entrances to the root canals may be sealed with IRM (Dentsply Caulk, Milford, DE, USA) (Fig. 6.41) and a base of glass ionomer cement is placed over the floor of the pulp chamber (Fig. 6.42).

As the downpack is carried out in one movement of the heated plugger, a continuous wave of heated GP is created, which is compacted apically and laterally down the root canal. This forces GP and sealer into the accessory anatomy of the root canal system (Fig. 6.43).

System B pluggers should never be heated to over 200°C and should never be activated in the root canal for longer than 2 seconds as this may result in thermal damage to the periodontal ligament. If the plugger fails to reach the desired length in the two second interval during the downpack, the plugger should be deactivated and apical pressure should be maintained for 10 seconds at the length obtained. Following this the plugger can be reactivated and the desired length should be reached easily.

Carrier-based systems

Carrier-based systems, e.g. Thermafil or Guttacore (Dentsply-Maillefer, Ballaigues, Switzerland), were designed to provide a quick and convenient method of filling the root canal system. They consist of an 'obturator', which is a solid but flexible plastic or cross-linked GP core, which is coated with GP (Fig. 6.44a). The function of the core is to carry the GP to the desired length. The GP coating is heated prior to placement in the root canal. Traditional Thermafil obturators are manufactured to correspond to the ISO standardized file tip sizes. These are colour coded in accordance with the ISO specifications. The taper of these carriers is 0.04 and will allow adequate filling of the root canals prepared with stainless steel and NiTi file systems. However, specific Thermafil

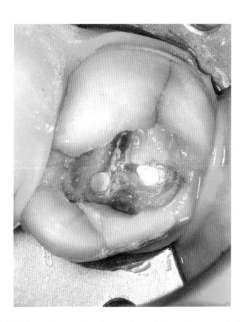

Figure 6.41 The entrances to the root canals have been sealed with increments of IRM (Dentsply Caulk, Milford, DE, USA) to prevent microbial recontamination of the filled root canals due to possible leaking coronal restorations.

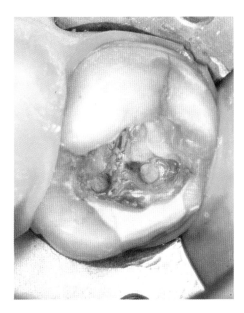

Figure 6.40 The coronal GP in the buccal root canals has been compacted to below the level of the cemento–enamel junction using endodontic pluggers.

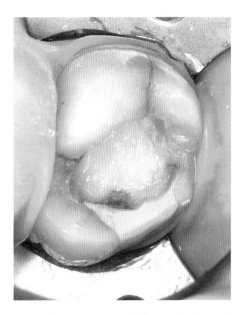

Figure 6.42 A glass ionomer cement (GIC) base has been placed over the floor of the pulp chamber.

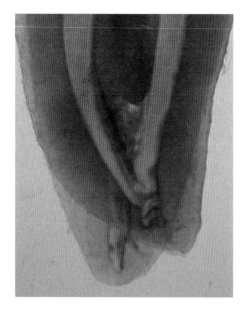

Figure 6.43 An endodontically treated, extracted molar tooth has been made transparent to demonstrate the quality of the root canal filling. Note that the isthmus between the mesial root canals has been filled with GP.

obturators have also been developed to correspond to the tip size and taper of specific NiTi file systems such as the ProTaper and GT systems (Dentsply-Maillefer, Ballaigues, Switzerland).

The following are the steps for successful root canal filling using the carrier-based system:

- The root canal is prepared to the desired length and apical diameter.
- A verifier is chosen which is the same size and taper as the corresponding master apical file. The verifier is introduced into the root canal to gauge the most appropriate obturator to use. The appropriate verifier should fit passively at the working length. The obturator corresponding to this verifier is chosen to fill the root canal (Fig. 6.44b).
- The root canal is dried and sealer is applied.
- A silicone stop on the chosen obturator is set to the working length. The obturator is placed in a specially designed oven, e.g. Thermaprep 2 oven (Dentsply-Maillefer, Ballaigues, Switzerland) (Fig. 6.44c), to heat the outer coating of GP.
- The obturator is now inserted in the root canal. Insertion should occur smoothly and without excessive force until the working length is reached.
- Firm apical pressure is maintained on the obturator handle for 1–2 minutes until the GP has cooled in order to counteract shrinkage of the material.
- The obturator handle can now be resected using a hot instrument or a specially designed, long shanked, round bur with a non-cutting surface. The friction created by this bur, used without water, sears off the handle.
- Specifically designed post preparation burs are available for use with this system.

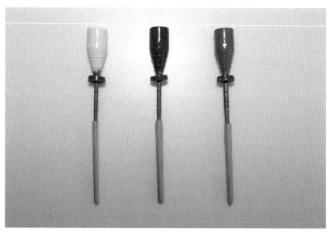

(a)

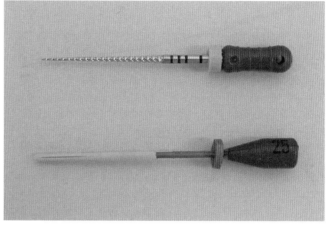

(b)

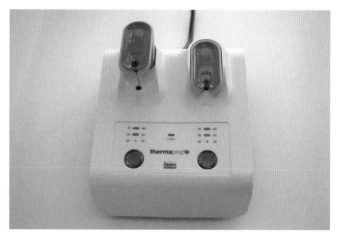

(c)

Figure 6.44 Thermafil (Dentsply-Maillefer, Ballaigues, Switzerland): (a) assorted range of Thermafil obturators; (b) Verifier (above) and the equivalent sized Thermafil obturator (below); (c) Thermaprep2 oven to heat the Thermafil obturators.

Master gutta-percha point placement troubleshooting

The clinician may encounter several problems when placing a master GP point. Table 6.4 summarizes the possible causes and various solutions to manage these problems.

Table 6.4 Master gutta-percha (GP) point placement troubleshooting

Problem	Possible causes	Solution
The master GP point will not reach the full working length	• The master GP point has a tip diameter larger than that of the prepared apical portion of the root canal	• Choose a master GP point with a tip diameter that corresponds to the prepared apical portion of the root canal. This can sometimes be achieved by choosing a GP point with a tip diameter smaller than the master apical file (MAF) diameter, and removing 0.5 mm increments from the tip until the tip diameter corresponds to the size of the apical preparation (recognized when tugback is achieved at the working length)
	• The master GP point has a taper greater than that of the prepared root canal	• This may happen when the root canal is prepared with stainless steel hand files and a GP point with a larger taper (designed for use with nickel-titanium (NiTi) files) is chosen as the master GP point. In these situations the tip diameter of the GP point may correspond to the prepared apical portion of the root canal but will be wider along its length and will bind coronally in the root canal before it reaches the full working length
	• The apical portion of the root canal is not prepared adequately to accommodate the master GP point	• Reintroduce the MAF and ensure it reaches the full working length easily. If it does not and a file with a smaller tip does, then re-prepare the apical portion of the root canal to the desired size
	• Dentinal chips may have blocked up the apical portion of the root canal and this may not have been noticed until now	• Use copious irrigation and small files (sizes 06, 08, 10, 15) to re-establish patency
	• Remnants from the coronal restoration (amalgam or composite debris) may have entered the root canal following late access cavity refinement	• This is unlikely to happen unless the access cavity is refined following preparation of the root canals. This should be avoided. The access cavity should be complete, at the latest, before the apical portion of the root canals are instrumented
		• If this is suspected, take a periapical radiograph of the tooth to confirm the presence of the filling material in the root canal and attempt to remove or bypass the dislodged material
I cannot achieve tugback at the working length	• The tip diameter of the master GP point is too small (this can happen even when the GP point corresponds to the MAF size)	• Choose a larger master GP point or trim the tip of the existing point by 0. 5 mm increments with a scalpel until tugback is achieved
		• If this fails the apical portion of the GP point can be customized to fit the apical portion of the prepared root canal (see 'Creation of a customized master GP point')
		• NB Tugback occurring at a length short of the working length may indicate inappropriate master point selection (too large) or that further preparation of the root canal is required

(continued)

Table 6.4 (*continued*)

Problem	Possible causes	Solution
When I insert the master GP point to the working length and remove it, it has buckled	• The tip diameter of the master point is too small and it is folding against the apical wall of the root canal instead of binding against the lateral walls	• See solutions for 'I cannot achieve tugback at the working length'
When I insert the master GP point to the working length and remove it the tip has bent back on itself	• The master point is being introduced into the root canal at the incorrect angle and is bending when it contacts the wall of the root canal. As the point is passed further into the root canal the tip bends back on itself further	• Align the GP point with the long axis of the root canal before introducing it into the root canal

Filling root canals with open apices

It may be necessary to carry out root canal treatment on teeth with open apices in the following situations:

- During normal tooth development the root of an immature tooth fails to form when the pulp of the affected tooth becomes necrotic, resulting in a blunderbuss apex.
- Resorption of the apical portion of the root of the tooth, for example, as a result of long-standing periapical periodontitis or pressure caused by an impacted tooth or a cyst.
- Overzealous mechanical preparation of the apical foramen may lead to loss of the natural apical constriction.

Regardless of the cause, it is challenging to fill these root canals. There is no resistance to apical movement of GP points due the absence of an apical taper associated with the root canal. The risk of extruding the root canal filling is therefore high and a well-sealing root canal filling is difficult to achieve. Several treatment options are available to overcome this problem all of which aim to provide a stop against which the root canal filling material can be packed. Historically, the root canal would be repeatedly dressed with calcium hydroxide over an extended period to stimulate the creation of an apical calcific barrier. The use of calcium silicate-based cements, (e.g. MTA), has largely superseded the other techniques as a method of creating an apical barrier in teeth with open apices. The material is based on Portland building cement and has been shown to be very biocompatible, with superior sealing qualities when used as a root canal filling material. The following provides a brief outline of how the material is applied (Fig. 6.45):

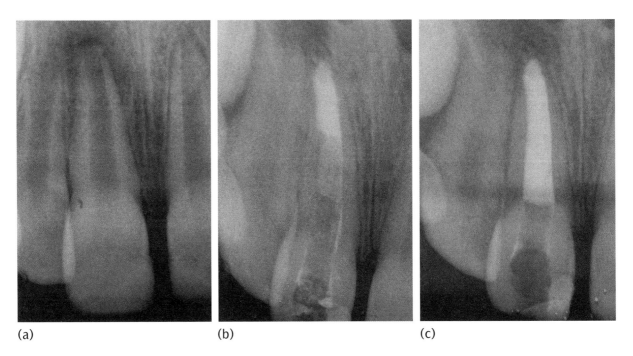

(a) (b) (c)

Figure 6.45 (a,b,c) Radiographs of a MTA apical plug in an immature permanent incisor tooth.

- The root canal is disinfected and dried.
- The calcium silicate-based cement is packed into the apical portion of the root canal using a carrier gun (Fig. 6.46) and premeasured endodontic pluggers. Ultrasonic tips can be used to vibrate the material into position. Enough material should be placed to provide an apical plug of 3–5 mm.
- The remainder of the root canal is then back-filled with heated GP and sealer to the cemento–enamel junction before a permanent coronal restoration is placed. It is no longer considered necessary to wait and check that the material has set prior to back-filling the root canal with GP.

This technique has some disadvantages:

- The material can be difficult to handle;
- A dental operating microscope is necessary for placement;
- Several control radiographs may be necessary to verify the accurate placement of the material.

These types of cases should be referred to an endodontist.

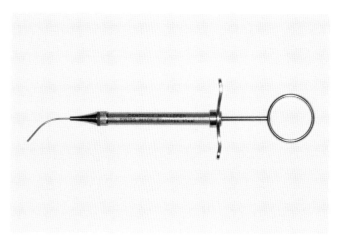

Figure 6.46 Calcium silicate cement gun: MAP System (Dentsply-Maillefer, Ballaigues, Switzerland).

Criteria for successful root canal filling

Regardless of the root canal filling technique used, the end result should be the same. The criteria for successful root canal filling are as follows:

- The entire working length should be filled;
- There should be no voids within the root canal filling;
- There should be no overextension of the root canal filling into the periapical tissues.

It should be remembered that success in these factors is dependent on the efficacy of the root canal preparation stage.

Summary points

- The objectives of root canal filling are to entomb any microbes remaining within the root canal system following preparation, and to seal all anatomical routes into the root canal system, thus preventing entry of nutritional sources or reinfection.
- There are many factors which may influence the time to fill the root canal. These include the preoperative status of the pulp, preoperative symptoms, the ability to disinfect and dry the root canal system, the procedural difficulty of a case, and patient related factors. Each tooth should be treated on a case-by-case basis.

- Various root canal filling materials are available. The most commonly used core material is gutta-percha (GP). An appropriate root canal sealer should be used in conjunction with the root canal core filling material.
- Various root canal filling techniques are available. These are broadly categorized into cold or warm compaction.
- Regardless of the material or technique used, the ideal root canal filling should extend from the root canal entrance to the apical constriction, and contain no voids.

Suggested further reading

American Association of Endodontics (2009) Obturation of root canal systems. *ENDODONTICS: Colleagues for Excellence Newsletter*, pp. 1–8. http://www.aae.org/.

Duncan HF and Kanagasingam S (2011) Section 4. Case 4.6. Obturation of the root canal system. In: Patel S and Duncan HF (eds) *Pitt Ford's Problem-Based Learning in Endodontology*, 1st edn, pp. 147–56. Chichester: Wiley-Blackwell.

Durack C and Patel S (2011) Section 8. Case 8.2. Internal root resorption. In: Patel S and Duncan HF (eds), *Pitt Ford's Problem-Based Learning in Endodontology*, 1st edn, pp. 296–302. Chichester: Wiley-Blackwell.

European Society of Endodontology (2006) Quality guidelines for endodontic treatment: consensus report of the European Society of Endodontology. *International Endodontic Journal* **39** 921–30.

Johnson WT and Kulild JC (2010) Obturation of the cleaned and shaped root canal system. In: Hargreaves KM, Cohen S and Berman LH (eds), *Pathways of the Pulp*, 10th edn, pp. 349–88. Missouri: Mosby Elsevier.

Patel S (2011) Section 3. Case 3.1. Apexification. In: Patel S and Duncan HF (eds), *Pitt Ford's Problem-Based Learning in Endodontology*, 1st edn, pp. 61–8. Chichester: Wiley-Blackwell.

Online Resource Centre

 To help you to develop and apply your knowledge and skills further, we have provided interactive learning resources online at http://www.oxfordtextbooks.co.uk/orc/patel/

7

Restoration of the endodontically treated tooth

Bhavin Bhuva and Francesco Mannocci

Chapter contents

Introduction

Microbes from the oral cavity are the main threat to the survival of the endodontically treated tooth. The coronal restoration (or seal), provides the first line of defence in preventing these microbes from potentially infecting the filled root canal system and ultimately causing inflammatory changes in the periapical tissues.

Apart from providing an optimum coronal seal, the definitive restoration must fulfil a number of further objectives (Table 7.1). Invariably, teeth requiring endodontics treatment are significantly compromised; therefore the definitive restoration will need to restore form, function, and aesthetic appearance. By establishing balanced occlusal contacts, over-eruption and tilting of the adjacent teeth can be prevented; whilst restoration of the contact areas will help to allow optimal health to be maintained in the supporting periodontal tissues, by reducing interproximal food impaction.

Table 7.1 The main objectives of treatment when restoring the endodontically treated tooth

- Provision of adequate coronal seal
- Protection of remaining tooth structure from fracture
- Re-establishing form (contact points)
- Restoring occlusal function
- Restoring aesthetics

Considerations when restoring endodontically treated teeth

How do endodontically treated teeth differ from vital teeth?

There is clear evidence that endodontically treated teeth are more susceptible to fracture than untreated teeth. It has been suggested that endodontically treated teeth may be weakened as a result of the biochemical and mechanical effects of endodontic treatment procedures on dentine. The use of irrigants (e.g. sodium hypochlorite (NaOCl)) and medicaments (e.g. calcium hydroxide) have been shown to alter the collagen structure and adversely affect the flexural strength and modulus of elasticity of dentine, making the tooth more susceptible to fracture.

Evidence would suggest that the loss of pulpal neurovascular supply does not appear to have a clinically significant effect on the mechanical properties of the remaining tooth structure. The most important factor that reduces the fracture resistance of endodontically treated teeth is the effect of cavity and root canal preparation procedures. Overzealous access cavity/post preparation and/or over-instrumentation of the root canal to an excessively wide taper must be avoided. The effects of loss of vitality and endodontic treatment procedures are listed in Table 7.2.

What factors will dictate whether a tooth is restorable?

When assessing a tooth that requires root canal treatment, the first consideration must be to determine whether it is possible to predictably restore the tooth following the completion of endodontic treatment, i.e. is the tooth restorable? This decision will be dictated by a number of factors, the most important being the extent of coronal tooth substance loss. In addition, the effect of the endodontic access cavity must also be considered. To evaluate the tooth it is necessary to remove the existing restoration and any associated caries, to determine the amount, position, and quality of remaining coronal dentine (Fig. 7.1). By removing the existing restoration it will

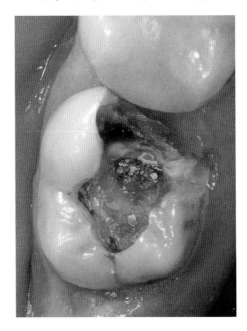

Figure 7.1 All the caries must be removed from this mandibular molar tooth before a decision can be made about its restorability.

Table 7.2 The effects of loss of vitality and endodontic treatment on a tooth

- Loss of tooth structure
- Dehydration of dentine
- Collagen alteration
- Effects of dismantling the coronal restoration
- Effects of irrigants and medicaments
- Loss of proprioception

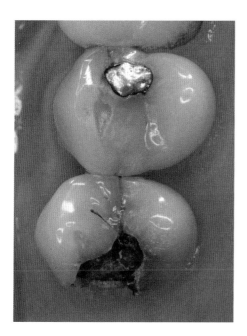

Figure 7.2 The carious maxillary second premolar tooth has both caries and a crack. Until the tooth is investigated, it will not be possible to make a definitive decision on the restorability of the tooth.

also be possible to exclude the presence of any cracks or undetected caries (Fig. 7.2).

What factors will influence the survival of the endodontically treated tooth?

There a very few robust studies assessing the longevity of endodontically treated teeth. One study has suggested that the probability of an endodontically treated tooth lasting 20 years is about 80 per cent.

The survival of a specific endodontically treated tooth will be influenced by a number of factors. These include the periodontal and restorative status of the tooth. A good coronal seal is an integral factor in ensuring the best possible lifespan for the endodontically treated tooth. There is also unequivocal evidence demonstrating that the survival of endodontically treated molar teeth is greatly enhanced by the placement of a cuspal coverage restoration. How well this restoration will last will be primarily dictated by the amount of remaining sound coronal tooth structure and, in particular, the ability to obtain an adequate ferrule effect. Teeth which lack sufficient dentine to obtain an adequate ferrule effect (see section 'What is the ferrule effect?'), particularly those restored with post-retained crowns, will be less likely to survive in the long-term.

Assuming the endodontically treated tooth has good periodontal health and sufficient remaining sound tooth structure, the most important factor dictating tooth longevity will be the endodontic prognosis. Effective cleaning and shaping of all root canals to full length, followed by high quality root canal filling will ensure the best chance of a favourable outcome. Other factors which may influence tooth survival will include occlusal considerations, whether the tooth is to be used as an abutment for a fixed or removable prosthesis.

What is the ferrule effect?

The ferrule effect is the collar of an extracoronal restoration (e.g. a crown) which encircles a circumferential ring of dentine (ideally of at least 2 mm in height) coronal to the preparation margins (Fig. 7.3). The presence of an adequate ferrule is critical to the predictable definitive restoration of a tooth. Without an adequate ferrule, undue stress is exerted on the core and/or post, leading to failure of the core or residual tooth substance (Fig. 7.4).

Deciding how to restore the endodontically treated tooth

There are a number of factors that must be considered when deciding how an endodontically treated tooth is best restored (Table 7.3). First and foremost, the amount of remaining tooth structure will be the most important consideration. When large amounts of tooth structure need to be replaced, the use of an adhesive material will permit the preservation of as much residual tooth tissue as possible. There is good evidence to show that the type of post-endodontic restoration required varies according to the tooth type. This is due to differences in both crown and root anatomy, as well as differences in the functional and non-functional forces encountered in different parts of the mouth.

Occlusion

The patient's occlusion will influence the restorative requirements of a tooth. For example, for a patient with canine disclusion in lateral excursive movements, it may not be necessary to protect the premolar units with cuspal coverage restorations. Conversely, in a patient exhibiting

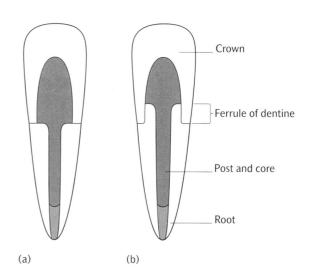

Figure 7.3 A diagrammatical representation of the ferrule effect (a) shows a post-retained crown with no ferrule whilst (b) shows the same restoration but this time with a collar of dentine coronal to the restorative margins. The presence of an adequate ferrule helps to prevent the transmission of undesirable forces through the post into the root.

Adapted from Patel S and Duncan H (2011) *Pitt Ford's Problem-Based Learning in Endodontology*. Printed with permission from Wiley-Blackwell.

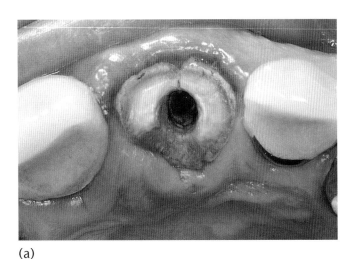

(a)

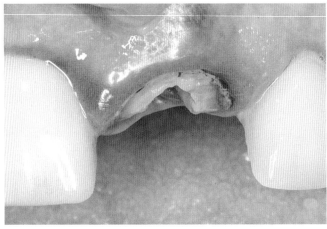

(b)

Figure 7.4 (a,b) The existing post crown has been lost from this maxillary central incisor tooth. There is insufficient sound coronal dentine available above the crown margins, and so a ferrule effect will not be achievable.

Table 7.3 Factors influencing the choice of definitive restoration for an endodontically treated tooth

- Amount of residual tooth structure
- Crown and root anatomy
- Location of tooth in arch
- Parafunction and other occlusal factors
- Bonding surface availability
- Moisture control
- Aesthetic considerations
- Patient preference
- Cost

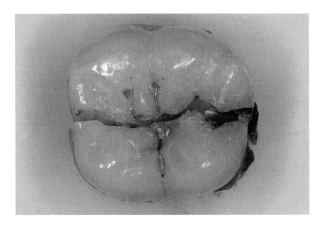

Figure 7.5 This unrestored mandibular molar tooth has fractured as a result of the patient's nocturnal grinding habit.

group function, the guiding units may require cuspal protection, even though the size of the restoration in itself does not necessarily warrant this.

A number of patients may have a nocturnal clenching or grinding habit. This is also known as parafunction. The forces generated during parafunctional events are significantly greater, and more prolonged than those encountered during mastication. Patients who parafunction may often report the fracture of restorations or teeth (Fig. 7.5). Careful examination may reveal cracked cusps or restorations, wear facets, or soft tissue signs of parafunction such as linea alba at the level of the occlusal plane or tongue ridging. Endodontically treated teeth with signs of parafunction should be restored with cuspal coverage restorations.

Aesthetic considerations

Patients are becoming increasingly dentally aware, and may have specific requests. This may be based on attitudes towards certain materials (e.g. amalgam) or purely due to aesthetic considerations (e.g. composite resin restorations or all ceramic crowns).

What is the best material to use for a core in an endodontically treated tooth?

The materials traditionally used for core placement in endodontically treated teeth are composite and amalgam. Composite materials, in addition to their aesthetic advantages have the added benefit of being adhesive and permit a more conservative cavity preparation than that required for amalgam restorations. Glass ionomer cement may also be used in certain situations. However, its use should be restricted to eliminating undercuts or space filling, as the material has very poor compressive strength. These materials have different attributes which must be evaluated so that the most appropriate material can be chosen for each specific clinical situation.

Do all endodontically treated teeth require crowns?

As discussed previously, endodontically treated teeth are more susceptible to fracture than untreated teeth (Fig. 7.6). Endodontically treated molar teeth, more often than not, require cuspal coverage protection. It

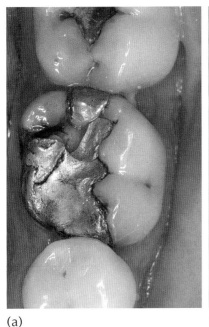
(a)

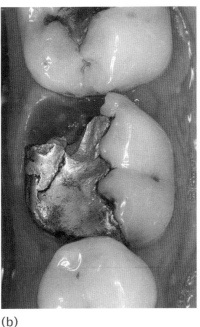
(b)

Figure 7.6 This endodontically treated mandibular molar tooth was restored with an amalgam restoration, but no cuspal coverage was provided. The patient declined to have a crown. (a) One year later, at a review appointment, it was noted that the disto-lingual cusp had fractured, and (b) following the removal of this, it was apparent that the tooth was unrestorable.

may often be possible to provide cuspal protection without the additional tooth substance loss incurred during full coverage crown preparation.

Restorations such as onlays (or partial coverage crowns) allow preservation of the axial walls of the tooth, and therefore unnecessary tooth tissue removal. The preparation of the buccal and/or lingual walls of a tooth for a full coverage preparation, may compromise the tooth structure such that there is little more than the core retaining the crown. This may lead to an early failure of the restoration. In these situations, an onlay may serve the purpose of protecting the residual tooth structure, but without the cost of weakening the tooth significantly.

Onlay restorations may be constructed in composite, ceramic, or gold. A further advantage of onlay restorations is that the margins are usually supragingival, allowing easier maintenance.

Anterior teeth

There appears to be little benefit in crowning endodontically treated incisors or canines unless there has been a considerable loss of tooth structure (e.g. both proximal surfaces in addition to the palatal access). The proportionate effect of tooth reduction during crown preparation is more significant in anterior teeth, particularly in the mandibular arch.

Crowns may occasionally be indicated for anterior teeth for purely aesthetic reasons. This may be the case when more conservative measures, such as internal bleaching, have not achieved the desired result (Fig. 7.7).

Premolar teeth

Following root canal treatment, premolars may require an indirect cuspal coverage if there is more than one marginal ridge involved in the restoration. However, premolar teeth also have relatively small crowns,

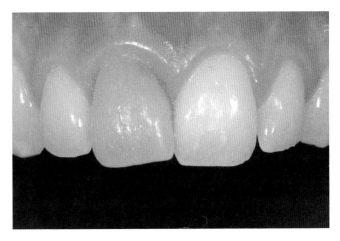

Figure 7.7 This non-vital maxillary central incisor tooth did not respond satisfactorily to internal bleaching. The tooth was subsequently crowned.

and the proportionate effect of crown preparation is again significant. Where appropriate, and when the occlusion permits, all-ceramic or composite partial crowns may be a more desirable option to preserve the maximum amount of coronal tooth structure. (Fig. 7.8).

Molar teeth

Endodontically treated molar teeth are the most susceptible to fracture and so cuspal protection with an indirect restoration is usually necessary (unless the restoration consists only of the endodontic access cavity). There are numerous studies that have demonstrated the superior

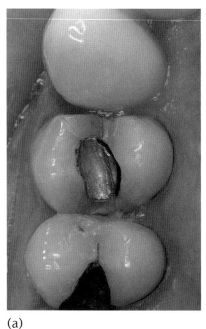

(a)

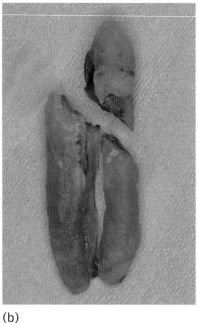

(b)

Figure 7.8 (a) This endodontically treated maxillary first premolar tooth has undergone a complex crown and root fracture. A number of fracture lines can be noted. (b) After the tooth was extracted the full extent of the fractures could be appreciated.

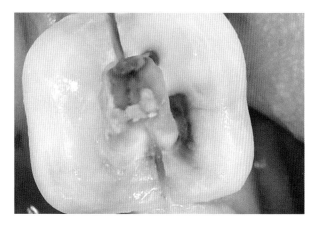

Figure 7.9 After removal of the coronal restoration and access into the pulp chamber it is apparent, utilizing magnification, that there is a complex fracture in this endodontically treated molar tooth.

Table 7.4 Factors that must be considered when a post is to be placed

- Amount of residual tooth structure—ferrule effect
- Suitable retention for core
- Root canal length
- Root canal curvature
- Root canal dentine thickness
- Occlusal factors

survival of molar teeth when an indirect cuspal coverage restoration has been placed after the endodontic treatment (Fig. 7.9).

In summary, although many endodontically treated teeth will require cuspal coverage protection, it is important to appreciate that the fulfilment of this objective should not be at the cost of unnecessary tooth preparation. Therefore, there may be situations where full coverage crown preparation is not necessary to protect an endodontically treated tooth.

What is the purpose of a post when restoring an endodontically treated tooth?

A post is required when there is insufficient remaining tooth structure to support a core. This situation will occur fairly frequently in compromised teeth. When deciding whether a post has to be placed, it is necessary to make a number of considerations (Table 7.4).

As a tooth requiring a post will almost always require cuspal coverage with an indirect restoration (e.g. a crown), it is important to consider what support the residual tooth structure will give for the core, as well as how much retention there will be for the restoration. Posts are more likely to be indicated in anterior teeth due to the relatively small crown size when compared with molar teeth. In fact, in molar teeth, even if the amount of residual coronal tooth structure is limited, the pulp chamber often offers sufficient retention for the core.

It is important to appreciate that posts do not reinforce teeth and therefore should not be used for this purpose. Posts transfer stresses into the root of the tooth. Axial forces tend to be distributed more favourably than lateral forces. Undesirable forces can be reduced by the presence of an adequate ferrule of dentine which will protect the root from being exposed to large lateral loads. Therefore, as with indirect cuspal coverage restorations, the longevity of teeth restored with posts appears to be dictated by the presence of an adequate ferrule.

Table 7.5 Factors influencing post performance

Factors	Effect	Relevance to post system
Ferrule of dentine	Predictability and longevity	Any
Length	More retention	Metal
Width	Little influence—adaptation more important	Any
Taper	Higher risk of root fracture—Parallel-sided posts perform better	Metal
Surface	Serrated posts	Metal
Material	Root fracture	Metal
	Decementation	Any
Water absorption	Failure of bonding	Fibre

It has been suggested that post length should be equal to or greater than the crown height. However, although optimizing post length is desirable, it is also important to preserve an adequate length of root canal filling material apically to prevent the persistence or development of apical periodontitis. At least 5 mm of apical root canal filling material should be preserved in order to maintain an adequate apical seal.

Post width does not appear to be as critical as post length, but it is important that the post is well-adapted to the root canal space, as the cement is the weakest link in the tooth-restoration complex. A number of characteristics have been studied in relation to the performance of posts. However, these attributes are relevant to metal post systems and less important for adhesive fibre post systems (Table 7.5).

What types of post are available?

There are many different types of post systems available, these can broadly be divided into direct or indirect post systems. A number of different designs and materials have been used for post fabrication (Table 7.6).

What is the best type of post?

Traditionally, indirect cast metal posts have been the most popular post technique when restoring compromised endodontically treated teeth. However, fibre posts have gained popularity as they appear to

have a number of additional advantages when compared with the cast post technique. Most fibre post systems are now made of quartz or glass fibres and are bonded adhesively within the root canal (Fig. 7.10).

A number of disadvantages have been suggested for metal post systems. The post space preparation for the cast post technique involves the removal of all undercuts, thus resulting in unnecessary removal of sound dentine. The most fundamental problem, however, is the lack of flexibility of metal posts. This applies to both direct and indirect post systems. Studies have demonstrated that root fractures are a recognized mode of failure that is more frequently associated with metal posts (Fig. 7.11). Failure is often terminal, necessitating extraction of the tooth.

Fibre posts seldom cause root fracture as they have a modulus of elasticity which is much closer to that of dentine. The failures associated with fibre post systems tend to be more retrievable. Fibre post-retained restorations most commonly fail due to post decementation,

Table 7.6 Posts according to material and type

Direct metal	Indirect metal	Direct non-metal
Stainless steel	Cast gold	Quartz
Titanium	Cast precious metal alloy	Glass
Gold	Cast non-precious metal alloy	Silica
		Carbon

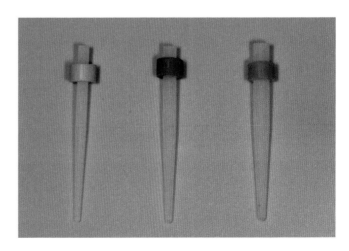

Figure 7.10 A selection of different sized fibre posts (RelyX Fiber Post, 3M Espe, St Paul, USA). Note that the posts have a tapered shape in the apical portion.

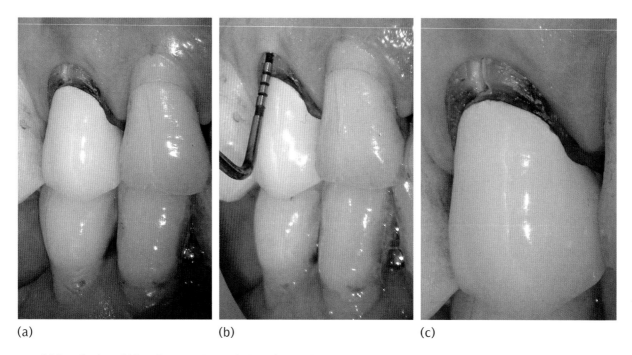

(a)   (b)   (c)

Figure 7.11 (a) Examination of this patient reveals a vertical root fracture in the maxillary first premolar tooth. The tooth has been restored with an indirect cast metal post crown. (b) There is an isolated increased probing depth associated with the fracture line. (c) Closer examination reveals separation of the fractured segments.

secondary caries, or chipping of the overlying composite restoration. The main cause for failure of fibre post systems is the ingress of moisture into the resin–dentine bonding interface during clinical function or thermocycling.

The performance of fibre posts has been shown to be equivalent to that of cast metal posts. Overall, the failure rate of fibre posts has been shown to be 7–11 per cent after 7–11 years of clinical service.

As for indirect cuspal coverage restorations, the survival of post-retained crowns appears to be most significantly influenced by the presence of an adequate ferrule irrespective of the type of post used. Therefore, although each post system has different advantages and disadvantages, ultimately, the survival of the restored tooth will be dictated by the amount of remaining coronal tooth structure.

Are there any problems associated with bonding in the root canal?

The use of adhesive materials within the root canal space presents a number of challenges. Firstly, following root canal treatment, there will often be remnants of gutta-percha (GP) and root canal sealer on the dentinal walls of the access cavity walls and/or post space. The physical presence of these materials will interfere with bonding non-specifically, whilst the use of certain materials, e.g. eugenol-containing sealers, will chemically inhibit the polymerization of composite materials. Therefore, great care must be taken to ensure the surface is adequately prepared for bonding.

A further problem with bonding is the anatomy of the root canal space itself. As there is a high ratio of bonded surface relative to unbonded

surface, the stresses created by polymerization shrinkage are unfavourable; this may lead to failure at the dentine-bonding interface.

The use of light polymerized materials within the root canal space is a further problem, as the curing lamp may not be able to transmit light adequately to all surfaces of the core or post preparation. The placement of a glass ionomer base may help to overcome the above problem (Fig. 7.12), the use of self-curing and dual-curing composites is also indicated.

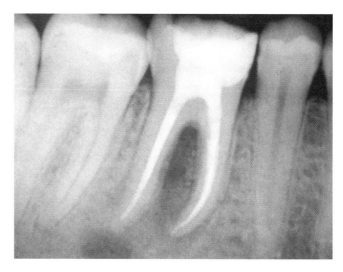

Figure 7.12 In this case, a base of glass ionomer cement (GIC) has been placed over the root canal filling. Composite resin has then been used to complete the core.

Foundation to clinical practice

The remainder of this chapter is concerned with the clinical aspects of restoring the endodontically treated tooth and aims to provide practical advice to help achieve the necessary treatment objectives.

When do we definitively restore the endodontically treated tooth?

The objectives of restoration following endodontic treatment were discussed earlier in the chapter. Included in these objectives were the provision of a good coronal seal, protection of the remaining tooth structure, and restoration of satisfactory aesthetics. It would therefore seem logical to satisfy these aims as soon as possible after the completion of the endodontic treatment. Leaving the tooth with an interim restoration for an extended period of time will leave it susceptible to fracture or microbial leakage. Molar teeth will be particularly susceptible to fracture. The risk increases further in teeth that are severely compromised or those which have existing fracture lines. In situations where the guidance in lateral or protrusive excursions involves the treated tooth there may be further indication for expedient protection.

If possible, the definitive core should be placed at the same appointment as the completion of endodontic treatment, whilst cuspal coverage with an indirect restoration should be provided within a few weeks of this; subject to the tooth being symptom-free.

Where there may be a delay in the placement of the final indirect cuspal coverage restoration it is important that the intermediate restoration provides adequate protection. For molar teeth, a cuspal coverage composite restoration or provisional crown may be appropriate. In most instances, three months may be an appropriate period of time to assess clinical healing (e.g. the resolution of a sinus tract or signs of improvement after a complex root canal retreatment). Guidelines suggest that radiographic healing can only be assessed after a minimum period of one year (see Chapter 8).

How do we prepare the endodontically treated tooth for restoration?

Following the completion of satisfactory endodontic treatment, the definitive restorative procedure must be planned.

When using adhesive materials, it is essential to ensure the complete removal of remnants of temporary and/or root canal filling materials from the access cavity. The use of magnification, e.g. loupes or a dental operating microscope, will greatly improve the visibility of remnants of root canal filling material in the access cavity. Removal may be carried out using a number of techniques, but the use of a dedicated endodontic ultrasonic tip, with copious water spray, is ideal. Specific ultrasonic tips designed for endodontic use allow unimpeded access of the pulp chamber and the root canal space itself, which is particularly useful when posts are to be adhesively bonded. The use of an ultrasonically activated tip will also minimize dentine removal when compared with a bur or post drill. Specifically designed microbrushes are also available to help in the cleaning of the root canal walls.

Cavity and root canal preparation will create a smear layer on the access cavity and root canal walls which will negatively affect the bonding of adhesive materials. Irrigation with ethylenediaminetetracetic acid (EDTA) solution subsequent to the completion of root canal preparation will assist in the removal of this. However, if for example, post preparation is then carried out, a new smear layer will be created. For removal of the smear layer, acid etching of dentine surfaces should be carried out with phosphoric acid. Acid etching may also help to get rid of persistent tags of GP or root canal sealer.

As mentioned previously, eugenol-containing endodontic and restorative materials may inhibit the polymerization of resin based materials. To overcome this, the root canal and access cavity can be rinsed with alcohol to sequester any free eugenol that may be present.

What are the practical considerations when using composite to restore the endodontically treated tooth?

It may be necessary to replace a significant volume of missing tooth tissue following endodontic treatment, particularly in molar teeth. Technical considerations may make the placement of an extensive composite restoration or core particularly demanding. In particular, it may be challenging to appropriately reconstruct the anatomical form of the tooth, particularly the contact areas, with direct adhesive materials. The following steps will assist in carrying out the procedure as predictably as possible.

Firstly, it is important to etch all available dentine surfaces, including the entrances to the root canals. It is desirable to use a fine microbrush

for this to ensure the etching agent is placed fully within the root canal entrance. Equally, the bonding agent should also be applied with a fine microbrush which is sufficiently small to place within the entrance to the root canal. Pooling of the bonding agent should be avoided and a paper point may be useful to soak up any excess. Pooling of bonding agent may predispose to incomplete curing or to the presence of voids between the restorative and root canal filling materials. Light-curing can then be carried out. There may be an issue with light transmission especially where the root canals are divergent or when the pulp chamber is

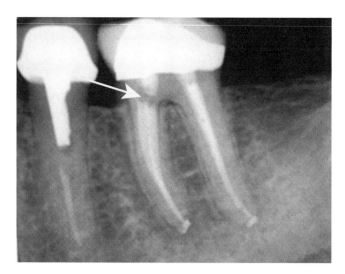

Figure 7.13 This composite core has not been placed satisfactorily. Voids (arrow) can be seen between the root canal filling material and core.

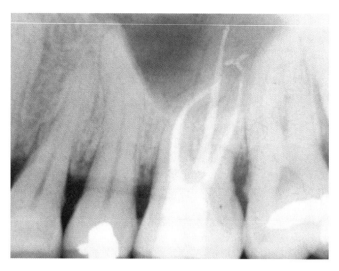

Figure 7.14 A composite core has been placed in this maxillary first molar tooth. A bulk-fill composite has been used to for the first increment.

deep. Therefore, it is important to ensure the bonding agent is cured on all surfaces prior to placement of the composite. Alternatively, the use of a chemical- or dual-cured bonding agent may be more appropriate.

For the reasons stated previously, it may occasionally be difficult to obtain complete curing of the composite resin placed into the root canals or deep into the pulp chamber. Initially, only a thin increment should be placed to ensure complete curing. Some bulk-fill composite materials are more translucent than conventional light cured composite materials, therefore permitting better light transmission through the entire thickness of the material. However, there is currently little data on the performance of these materials.

When using a conventional hybrid composite it may be challenging to get the restorative material to adapt closely to the root canal filling, resulting in voids between the core and root canal filling (Fig. 7.13). Occasionally, the material may be difficult to pack into the entrance of the root canal; instead it may stick to the plugger. One possible cause for this is incomplete curing of the bonding resin.

A large clean endodontic plugger may assist with the placement of the first few increments of composite. Extraneous light from adjunctive light sources (loupes or dental operating microscope) should be excluded using an appropriate filter to avoid premature curing of light-cure materials.

Recent developments have led to a number of novel bulk-fill flowable composite materials. These materials are designed to allow the quick build-up of large restorations and cores. Bulk-fill composites can be placed more easily and with much less contraction shrinkage than conventional composite materials. As previously mentioned, modern bulk-fill materials are also more translucent than conventional composites, facilitating more effective light-curing (Fig. 7.14).

A new group of composite materials known as *siloranes* have recently been developed. Siloranes have a unique ring-opening polymerization chemistry, which results in almost negligible shrinkage. These materials are an exciting prospect for the restoration of endodontically treated teeth. Excellent isolation is imperative when utilizing silorane materials.

What are the differences in restoring anterior and posterior teeth?

In general, endodontically treated teeth will either be definitively restored with a direct plastic or indirect restoration. As discussed earlier in the chapter, a plastic restoration (e.g. composite resin restoration) may often be appropriate for anterior teeth, whilst indirect restorations will usually be the restoration of choice for endodontically treated posterior teeth.

Anterior teeth

Direct restorations for anterior teeth

Composite restorations and core materials

Where an endodontically treated anterior tooth has only undergone moderate tooth tissue loss, definitive restoration with composite resin will invariably be the treatment of choice.

Modern resin-bonding and composite materials will provide satisfactory aesthetics in most situations. In order to achieve an optimal aesthetic result it is imperative to ensure that all residual root canal filling materials and/or sealer have been removed from the bonding surface prior to restoration. In addition to compromising bonding, residual root canal filling materials may also affect the final aesthetic result. The use of composite is also preferable for core build-up when an all-ceramic or indirect composite restoration is planned.

Restorative procedures should ideally be carried out under rubber dam isolation. When restoring the proximal areas of the tooth it is necessary to also isolate the neighbouring teeth. A shade should be taken prior to rubber dam isolation, i.e. before the dentine becomes dehydrated. If internal bleaching has been carried out it has been suggested that subsequent bonding may be affected temporarily by oxidizing products produced by the bleaching agent. It has therefore been recommended that definitive restoration with an adhesive material should be deferred for at least two weeks after bleaching.

It is important to ensure that the coronal level of the root canal filling material is kept below the cemento–enamel junction in order to avoid compromising the appearance of the definitively restored tooth. This is also the case when internal bleaching procedures are to be carried out.

Indirect restorations for anterior teeth

Veneers
As endodontically treated anterior teeth will invariably have been accessed from the palatal surface, the justification for providing a ceramic laminate veneer rather than a full-coverage crown for conservation reasons would appear invalid. From the perspective of tooth preservation, the advantages of a veneer may be even less relevant due to the development of newer materials for all-ceramic crowns; these require less axial reduction but perform well under clinical function.

A direct composite veneer may be a pragmatic approach when the result obtained from internal bleaching is unsatisfactory and a conservative solution is required. Minimal, if any, tooth reduction should be performed.

Metal-ceramic crowns
A crown may be required for the restoration of an endodontically treated anterior tooth when there has been significant loss of tooth structure or where conservative aesthetic treatment measures (e.g. internal bleaching) have been unsuccessful in achieving a satisfactory aesthetic result.

Metal-ceramic crowns are the usual choice when an indirect restoration is indicated for an anterior tooth. However, it must be acknowledged that the preparation for a metal-ceramic restoration requires significant reduction of the buccal (and other) surfaces of the tooth (approximately 1.8–2 mm). The amount of axial reduction may therefore significantly compromise the strength of the remaining tooth structure. With this in mind, consideration of the effect of crown preparation on the residual tooth tissue must be made.

Metal-ceramic crowns may be indicated in those situations where the tooth to be restored has a metallic core or post that precludes the use of a translucent all-ceramic restoration. These restorations may also be useful when the residual tooth structure has discoloured significantly and needs to be masked.

Gold-porcelain infusion crowns
Gold-porcelain infused indirect restorations have two advantages over conventional metal-ceramic restorations. Firstly, the buccal tooth reduction required for these restorations is 1–1.2 mm. This is considerably less than that needed for a conventional metal-ceramic crown preparation. Secondly, the colour of the underlying gold allows a superior aesthetic result, particularly in the cervical area of the restoration. Here, the use of a conventional metal-ceramic restoration may sometimes result in a discoloured marginal appearance.

All-ceramic crowns
All-ceramic crowns are increasingly being recommended as viable restorations for both anterior and posterior teeth. Modern all-ceramic materials have sufficient strength in thin section to withstand the forces imparted during normal clinical function. When used in conjunction with tooth-coloured post and core materials, their aesthetics are far superior to those achievable with conventional metal-ceramic units. The aesthetic advantage of these restorations is most evident in the marginal areas closest to the soft tissues, and also at the incisal edge, where some translucency may often be desirable. As discussed previously, the benefit of reduced axial tooth reduction is greatest for anterior teeth (Fig. 7.15).

Posterior teeth

Direct restorations and core materials for posterior teeth

Amalgam restorations and cores
Conventional amalgam restorations that include an interproximal extension, but which do not provide cuspal coverage cannot be considered as long-term definitive restorations for endodontically treated molar teeth; due to the high risk of crown or root fracture. Therefore, where possible, amalgam restorations should be designed with at least 2 mm cuspal coverage. Cuspal coverage amalgam restorations may be suitable as interim restorations for mandibular molars, but are aesthetically poor and so they may not be as appropriate for maxillary molar teeth.

When restoring endodontically treated maxillary molars, the functional palatal cusp should always be protected; coverage of the buccal cusps may not be necessary, particularly if there are no deflective contacts in lateral excursive movements. When restoring mandibular molars, all cusps should be protected.

Amalgam is still commonly used as a core material prior to the cuspal coverage of posterior teeth. The Nayyar core technique has been suggested when using amalgam as a core material in endodontically treated teeth. The technique involves the removal of 2–4 mm of coronal gutta-percha from each root canal; it would appear desirable to remove the root canal filling material with a heated instrument rather than by mechanical means. If rotary instruments are used to remove the coronal portion of root canal filling (e.g. Gates Glidden drills) then great care must be taken to avoid the unnecessary removal of dentine, particularly in the furcal region of molar teeth. Excessive dentine removal may lead to strip perforation of the root.

Following compaction of the coronal portion of root canal filling material at the appropriate level, the amalgam is then packed into the entrance to the root canals; an endodontic plugger is the most appropriate instrument to carry this out. The natural divergence of the root canals and undercuts found in the pulp chamber provide retention for the coronal-radicular dowel and core. The amalgam in the pulp chamber offers resistance to both horizontal and vertical forces (Fig. 7.16).

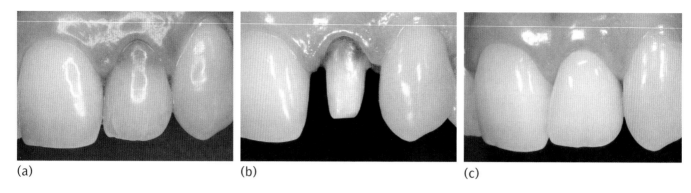

(a) (b) (c)

Figure 7.15 (a) Following endodontic treatment this discoloured maxillary lateral incisor tooth cannot be satisfactorily restored with a plastic restoration. (b) The tooth is prepared for an all-ceramic crown. (c) The crown is definitively cemented with an adhesive material.

Adapted from Mannocci F, Cavalli G and Gagliani M (2008) *Adhesive Restoration of Endodontically Treated Teeth*. Printed with permission from Quintessence Publishing.

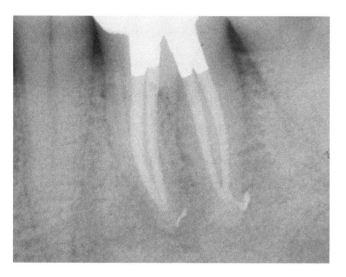

Figure 7.16 An amalgam Nayyar core has been placed following the completion of endodontic treatment of this mandibular first molar tooth.

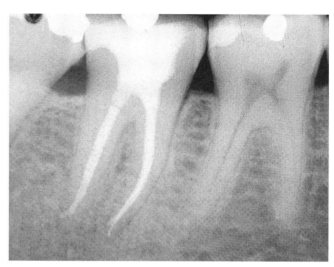

Figure 7.17 A composite core has been placed following endodontic retreatment of this mandibular first molar tooth.

Composite resin restorations and cores

In general, composite resin restorations cannot be regarded as long-term definitive restorations in functional endodontically treated posterior teeth. The exception to this may be when there has only been a minimal loss of tooth structure and both marginal ridges remain intact (Fig. 7.17).

When restoring endodontically treated teeth, the loss of tooth structure caused by caries and the access cavity preparation may make the placement of extensive direct composite resin restorations more challenging. In particular, where tooth substance loss is considerable, it may be difficult to satisfactorily reconstruct the anatomical form of the tooth, in particular the contact areas of molar teeth. The provision of large direct composite restorations may be

further complicated if cuspal coverage needs to be incorporated into the restoration. There is no consensus on the minimum thickness of composite resin that is required to protect the cusps of endodontically treated teeth from fracture, but a minimum of 2–3 mm would seem sensible.

It is always desirable to place composite restorations under rubber dam isolation. It may be necessary to isolate several teeth when restoration of the proximal areas of a tooth is required. Floss ligatures may be useful in securing the dam so that it does not impinge on the contact areas of the tooth being restored. It is imperative to use an appropriate matrix to allow proper adaptation of the restorative material in the contact areas. Ideally, where a metal band is to be used, the contact areas should be wedged and then burnished to provide optimal approximation (Fig. 7.18).

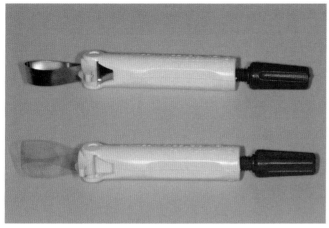

(a)

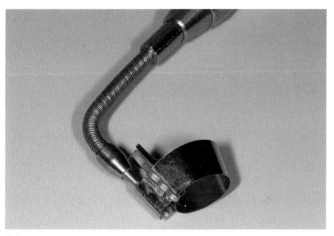

(b)

Figure 7.18 A number of disposable matrix bands are now available in the marketplace. Examples include the (a) Omni-Matrix system (Ultradent Products, South Jordan, UT, USA) and the (b) AutoMatrix (Dentsply, Addlestone, United Kingdom).

The placement of composite resin into the entrance to the root canals may be greatly enhanced by using an endodontic plugger, assisted by the use of an operating microscope or loupes. The use of a chemical- or dual-cured composite material may overcome the problem of inadequate light transmission within divergent root canals.

Indirect restorations for posterior teeth

The importance of placing a full-coverage indirect restoration on an endodontically treated molar tooth is based on studies demonstrating that tooth survival is significantly enhanced following the placement of cuspal coverage restorations. It is the author's opinion that inlays or partial cuspal coverage restorations are not, in general, appropriate for endodontically treated posterior teeth.

Gold onlays

Endodontically treated posterior teeth are often severely compromised and therefore gold onlays may offer the most conservative treatment as the preparation may be customized to permit the optimal preservation of residual tooth structure (Fig. 7.19).

The reduction required for indirect gold restorations may be as little as 0.7 mm, on non-functional surfaces, whilst as much as 1.5 mm may be required for the functional cusps. Gold onlays may be particularly useful when there is limited interocclusal space. Although gold onlays are not aesthetic restorations, they are still appropriate for most endodontically treated posterior teeth. If a gold onlay restoration is planned, full coverage of all of the cusps is usually advisable. Gold onlays may be particularly useful in patients who parafunction; as porcelain is more abrasive when the restoration is opposed by a natural tooth.

Gold crowns

Like gold onlays, gold crowns are only appropriate in teeth where aesthetics are not a concern. Full-coverage indirect gold restorations permit the preservation of a greater amount of sound tooth structure when compared to metal-ceramic crowns, as substantially less tooth reduction is required. The amount of reduction required during preparation is similar to that described for gold onlays.

Composite resin onlays and crowns

A direct, self- or dual-cure composite resin core is usually placed prior to the provision of a composite resin onlay or crown. Ideally, the shade of the core should be different to that of the surrounding dentine so that it is possible to differentiate the restorative material. The core acts as a guide during preparation of the indirect restoration.

Indirect composite restorations are usually light-curable microceramic composite resins. Indirect composite materials generally have higher fracture resistance than direct conventional or hybrid composites. However, they are not more resistant to fracture than all-ceramic units. Variations in the survival of direct and indirect composites have been attributed to the difference in adhesive strengths achieved with direct bonding when compared with those obtained with the use of a cement lute.

The onlay preparation for indirect composite resin or all-ceramic material requires a minimum tooth reduction of 1.5–2 mm. The margins recommended for these preparations are normally a 90° shoulder finish whilst the internal line angles of the cavity should be rounded. Proximal boxes must be extended apical to the contact points and internal walls should be divergent to avoid undercuts in the preparation. Coverage of all cusps with a thickness of approximately 2.5–3 mm is usually recommended.

Glass ionomer cement or flowable composite resin may be placed over the root canal filling material in order to achieve the required thickness and internal cavity form for the preparation. Indirect composite

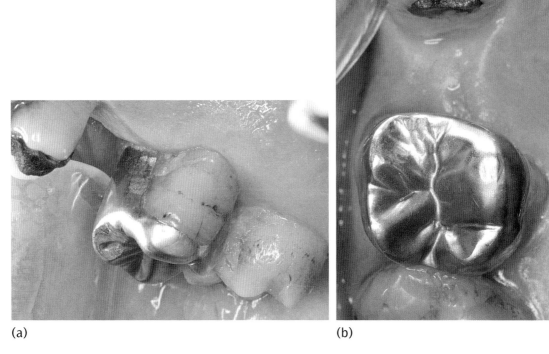

(a)   (b)

Figure 7.19 (a,b) This endodontically treated maxillary molar tooth has been restored with a gold onlay restoration. This restoration has permitted maximum preservation of the remaining tooth tissue.

and ceramic restorations are usually cemented with adhesive resin cements; cementation should ideally be carried out under rubber dam isolation (Fig. 7.20).

All-ceramic crowns

As previously discussed, there are numerous systems available for the manufacture of all-ceramic restorations. Over a five year observation period, it would appear that the survival of posterior all-ceramic crowns is equivalent to that of metal-ceramic units. However, all-ceramic restorations may not be the ideal choice for restoring endodontically treated posterior teeth in patients who parafunction.

Metal-ceramic crowns

Metal-ceramic units are the most frequently chosen indirect restoration for endodontically treated posterior teeth. As previously discussed, a disadvantage of metal ceramic restorations is that they require substantially greater tooth reduction in order to create sufficient space for both metal and porcelain materials (Fig. 7.21).

When is a post required?

The factors that must be considered when deciding on the suitability of a tooth for post placement are listed in an earlier part of this chapter (Table 7.4). As discussed previously, post placement is indicated if the amount of residual tooth structure is insufficient to retain a core. However, irrespective of whether a post is to be used or not, the presence of an adequate ferrule has been shown to be the most important factor in determining the performance of indirect cuspal coverage restorations (Fig. 7.22).

Under dynamic functional loading, posts will exert stresses along the root, which can potentially lead to root fracture. Where there is at least a 2 mm circumferential ring of dentine coronal to the margin of the crown preparation, the effect of these forces is somewhat protected from being transmitted unfavourably to the root.

In situations where it is not possible to obtain an adequate ferrule, it may be necessary to consider crown lengthening or orthodontic extrusion of the tooth. These treatment measures will also allow the restorative margins to be placed at a cleansable level and without them impinging on the biological width (Fig. 7.23).

Wherever possible, post preparation and placement should be carried out under rubber dam isolation. A split dam technique may be useful in these circumstances. Furthermore, where an indirect post is being constructed, it is important to provide a good coronal seal in the interim.

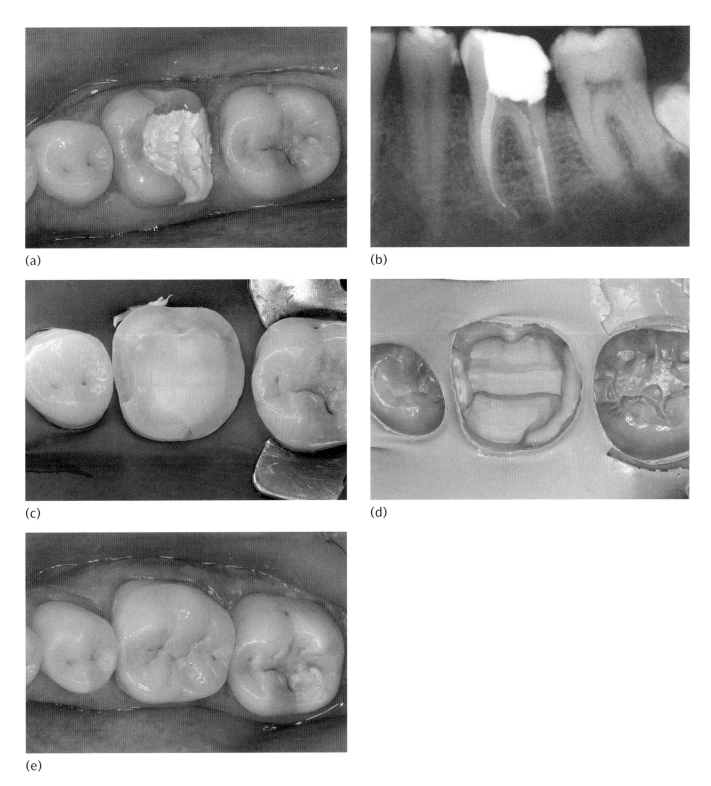

(a)

(b)

(c)

(d)

(e)

Figure 7.20 (a,b) This endodontically treated mandibular first molar tooth requires cuspal coverage. As there is still a good amount of sound tooth structure it is decided that a full coverage crown is not required. (c,d) Following placement of the core, the tooth is prepared for a full coverage composite onlay. (e) The completed restoration is cemented with a resin luting cement.

Adapted from Mannocci F, Cavalli G and Gagliani M (2008) *Adhesive Restoration of Endodontically Treated Teeth.* Printed with permission from Quintessence Publishing.

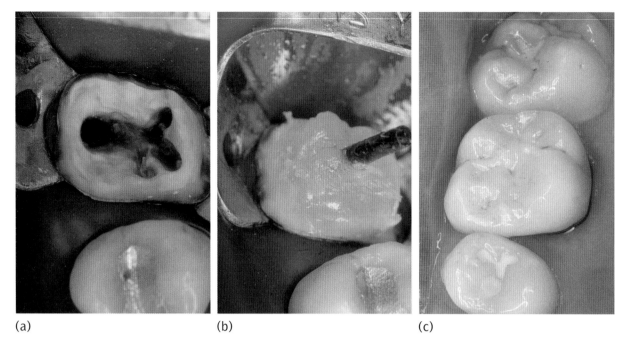

(a)   (b)   (c)

Figure 7.21 (a) This compromised maxillary first molar tooth requires reconstruction following root canal treatment. (b) A fibre post and composite core have been placed. (c) The final metal-ceramic crown is cemented.

Adapted from Mannocci F, Cavalli G and Gagliani M (2008) *Adhesive Restoration of Endodontically Treated Teeth*. Printed with permission from Quintessence Publishing.

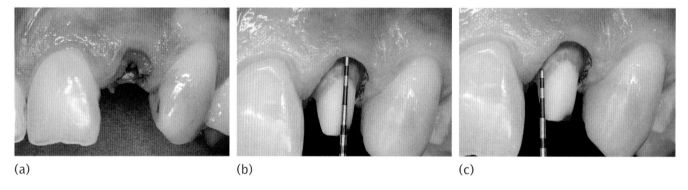

(a)   (b)   (c)

Figure 7.22 (a,b,c) Even in this significantly compromised maxillary lateral incisor tooth it has been possible to obtain a ferrule of 3 mm of dentine. Ideally, the ferrule of dentine should be available on all surfaces of the tooth.

Adapted from Mannocci F, Cavalli G and Gagliani M (2008) *Adhesive Restoration of Endodontically Treated Teeth*. Printed with permission from Quintessence Publishing.

Indirect posts

Posts may be either direct or indirect. Indirect posts are usually fabricated cast metal posts which can either be constructed from an acrylic pattern which is built up directly in the mouth (Fig. 7.24), or more usually constructed from an impression of the completed post space and crown preparation.

When preparing a tooth for an indirect cast metal post it is imperative to ensure that all undercuts have been removed and that any thin sections of unsupported dentine have been eliminated. Preparation is usually carried out using a dedicated post preparation kit which offers standardized sizes of drill and corresponding impression and temporary posts (Fig. 7.25). It is important to ensure that the post space preparation is clear of unwanted root canal filling material and debris at the time of impression taking and post cementation.

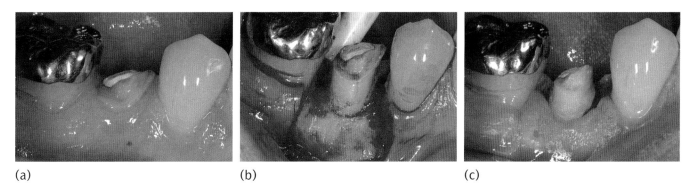

(a)   (b)   (c)

Figure 7.23 Crown lengthening has been used to obtain an adequate ferrule effect. (a) Prior to treatment, there is insufficient tooth structure to retain an indirect restoration. (b) Following, reflection of a flap, the bone level has been moved apically and recontoured. (c) The completed procedure has provided a further 2–3 mm of dentine for the placement of the final restoration.

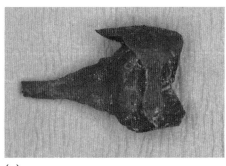

(a)

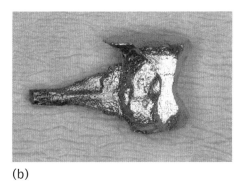

(b)

Figure 7.24 (a,b) A direct acrylic (Duralay) pattern is used to produce the finished cast post and core. Alternatively, an impression of the preparation and tooth can be taken.

Direct (pre-fabricated) posts

Metal Posts

Most contemporary direct metal post systems are of a serrated or threaded parallel-sided design. Commonly, these posts are constructed from titanium or stainless-steel alloys. Parallel-sided serrated posts have been shown to be more retentive, yet less likely to cause root fracture than tapered smooth posts. Metal posts may be adhesively cemented after which a direct composite core can then be built-up. The principles for the use of direct metal posts are the same as those indicated for fibre posts.

Fibre posts

There are a number of complete fibre post systems available in the market place (Fig. 7.26). The survival rate of teeth restored with indirect metal posts appears to be similar to those restored with pre-fabricated fibre posts, composite cores, and crowns.

When using a fibre post system, post preparation and cementation may be carried out at the same time as the endodontic treatment. There are several advantages to this:

- The orientation and anatomy of the root canal is clearly known, and therefore the risk of an iatrogenic accident during post preparation is minimized.

- Placing the post immediately after the completion of endodontic treatment reduces microleakage into the root canal space by sealing the root canal coronally, and also by preventing the need for a temporary post crown, which may either leak and/or decement.

- Reduces the number of visits and overall treatment time, by allowing crown preparation to be carried out at the same visit as the endodontic treatment.

However, caution must be exercised when using rubber dam during post preparation, as it may be difficult to orientate the tooth correctly, potentially leading to the misdirected use of rotary instruments within the root canal. This may be of particular relevance with teeth which are severely rotated or tilted.

The clinical sequence for the placement of a fibre post-retained composite core (see Fig. 7.27) is as follows:

1. *Post space preparation*: ideally, preparation of the root canal should be minimal. The unnecessary removal of dentine associated with the use of post drills will result in thinning of the root canal walls, weakening the tooth considerably.

2. *Preparation of root canal dentine*: rotary instruments such as Gates Glidden or Largo drills may be useful for removing GP; ultrasonic instruments used with magnification may also be used for this purpose. The root canal can be rinsed with alcohol if a eugenol-based sealer has been used during the root canal treatment.

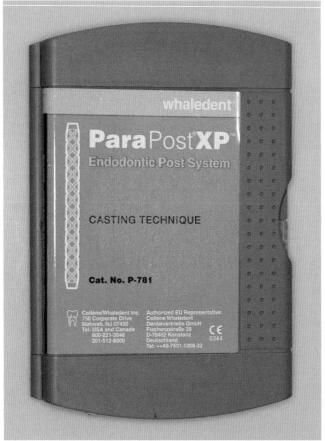

(a)

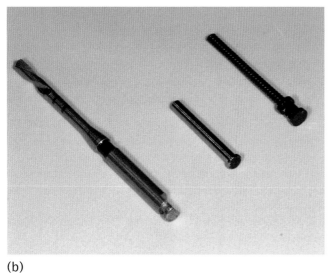

(b)

Figure 7.25 (a) An example of a post preparation system (ParaPost XP, Coltène Whaledent XP, Altstätten, Switzerland). (b) The drills are provided with corresponding temporary and impression posts.

(a)

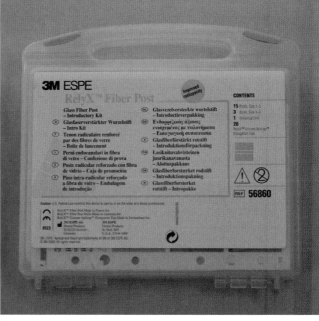

(b)

Figure 7.26 Examples of fibre post systems: (a) ParaPost Fiber White (Coltène Whaledent XP, Altstätten, Switzerland) and (b) RelyX Fiber Post (3M Espe, St Paul, USA).

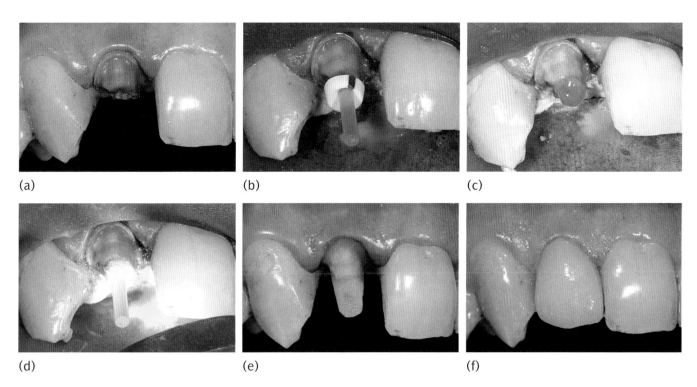

(a) (b) (c)

(d) (e) (f)

Figure 7.27 (a) Following removal of the existing crown and caries, the restorability of the residual tooth structure was assessed and it was apparent that an adequate ferrule effect could be achieved. Root canal retreatment of the tooth was completed. (b) After choosing the appropriate post, (c) the root canal space was etched, washed, and dried. (d) The cement was light cured, after which a composite core was built up. (e) The crown preparation was completed and (f) subsequently restored with an all-ceramic crown.

Adapted from Patel S and Duncan H (2011) *Pitt Ford's Problem-Based Learning in Endodontology*. Printed with permission from Wiley-Blackwell.

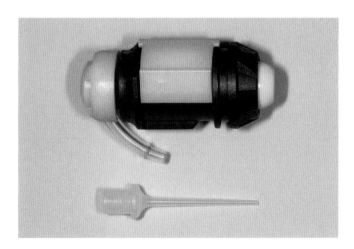

Figure 7.28 An example of a resin cement which can be used to adhesively bond fibre posts. Rely X Unicem (3M Espe, St Paul, USA) is provided with a delivery tip which aids in the delivery of the cement into the post space.

3. *Bonding to root canal dentine*: the chosen fibre post should be cemented with either a chemical- or dual-cured resin cement; usually prior etching of the root canal dentine is required. Paper points may be used to ensure that the root canal space is adequately dried. Dentine bonding agents should be used if a composite cement is being used to lute the post. A long thin microbrush can be used to aid application. Paper points can be used to avoid pooling of the bonding agent. Light curing can then be completed. Today, many self-etching adhesive cements are available for the cementation of fibre posts.

4. *Preparation of post for bonding*: if the post has been checked in the root canal prior to cementation, the surface of the post should be cleaned with alcohol after which bonding agent can be applied to the surface and lightly air dried. Silanization of the post has also been advocated.

5. *Post cementation*: the chosen cement can be injected into the root canal using a specially designed tip that facilitates delivery to the base of the post space (Fig 7.28). The use of a specific delivery tip ensures that the post cement fills the entire space, preventing air void formation. The selected post should then be inserted into the root canal to the desired length. Agitation of the post should be avoided to minimize air inclusion. If necessary, the material should then be light-cured, ensuring that the post is held *in situ* during the curing process.

6. *Core build-up:* the remainder of the core can then be built up with the same dual-cure composite used to cement the post, or alternatively a conventional light-cure composite may be used. It is important to ensure that the entire post is covered in composite to prevent moisture absorption into the post-core complex. If the post needs to be reduced in length his should be done with a diamond disc under copious water spray prior to core build-up.

7. *Crown preparation*: may be carried out at the same visit.

Summary points

- There are a number of objectives which must be fulfilled when restoring the endodontically treated tooth. These include:
  - Providing an adequate coronal seal;
  - Protection of remaining tooth structure from fracturing;
  - Re-establishing form, in particular the contact areas;
  - Restoring occlusal function;
  - Restoring aesthetics.
- The assessment of the endodontically treated tooth can only be made once the tooth has been fully disassembled, i.e. all restorative materials and caries have been removed. The effect of the endodontic access cavity must be considered, as must the location and extent of any cracks.
- The restorative requirements for the endodontically treated tooth are influenced by a number of factors which include location in the mouth, remaining coronal tooth structure, occlusion and aesthetic requirements.
- Numerous studies have demonstrated the superior survival of molar teeth when an indirect cuspal coverage restoration has been placed after the completion of endodontic treatment. Evidence has also demonstrated that there does not appear to be any advantage in crowning endodontically treated anterior teeth.
- The predictability of any indirect cuspal coverage restoration appears to be related to the ability to achieve an adequate ferrule effect. The ferrule can be defined as the collar of sound dentine (of adequate height and thickness) coronal to the preparation margins.
- A post is required when there is not enough tooth structure to support a core. This situation will occur fairly frequently in compromised teeth. When deciding whether a post has to be placed, it is necessary to make a number of considerations. Posts are more commonly indicated in anterior teeth.
- The use of modern adhesive materials facilitates the placement of both cores and posts in endodontically treated teeth in such a way that the remaining tooth structure can be optimally conserved and the tooth can be restored as aesthetically as possible.
- There is increasing evidence to support the use of fibre posts when restoring very compromised endodontically treated teeth. Fibre posts would appear to perform as well as both direct and indirect metal posts yet the modes of failure appear to be more retrievable.

Suggested further reading

Ferrari M, Cagidiaco MC, Goracci C, Vichi A, Mason PN, Radovic I and Tay F (2007) Long-term retrospective study of the clinical performance of fiber posts. *American Journal of Dentistry* **20**, 287–91.

Mannocci F and Cavalli G (2008) Fibre posts. In: Mannocci F, Cavalli G and Gagliani M (eds) *Adhesive restoration of endodontically treated teeth*, pp. 73–8. London: Quintessence Publishing.

Nayyar A, Walton RE and Leonard LA (1980) An amalgam coronal-radicular dowel and core technique for endodontically treated posterior teeth. *Journal of Prosthetic Dentistry*. **43**, 511–15.

Schillingburg HT, Jacobi R and Brackett SE (1987) *Fundamentals of tooth preparations for cast metal and porcelain restorations*. Chicago: Quintessence.

Sorensen JA and Engelman MJ (1990) Ferrule design and fracture resistance of endodontically treated teeth. *Journal of Prosthetic Dentistry* **63**, 529–36.

Sorensen JA and Martinoff JT (1984) Intracoronal reinforcement and coronal coverage: a study of endodontically treated teeth. *Journal of Prosthetic Dentistry* **51**, 780–4.

Stankiewicz NR and Wilson PR (2002) The ferrule effect: a literature review. *International Endodontic Journal* **35**, 575–81.

Online Resource Centre

 To help you to develop and apply your knowledge and skills further, we have provided interactive learning resources online at http://www.oxfordtextbooks.co.uk/orc/patel/

8
Treatment outcomes

*Justin J. Barnes
and Shanon Patel*

Chapter contents

Introduction

This chapter will introduce the underlying theory of treatment outcomes before exploring how this transfers to clinical practice. It is important that you read the whole chapter to understand how the theory and practice of treatment outcomes are related.

What is meant by the outcome of endodontic treatment?

The aim of endodontic treatment is to prevent or cure periapical periodontitis. When assessing the outcome of endodontic treatment, we are essentially assessing whether we have been able to meet this aim. The ideal outcome is, therefore, the absence, or in cases where there were signs of preoperative periapical periodontitis, the resolution of periapical periodontitis after endodontic treatment. In some cases, there will be emergence, persistence, or recurrence of periapical periodontitis after endodontic treatment.

There are several ways to measure and categorize the outcome of endodontic treatment. These can be broadly categorized into:

- *Strict/stringent criteria*. This requires no symptoms, no clinical signs of disease, and no periapical radiolucencies for endodontic treatment to be deemed a success (Fig. 8.1a,b). This is the ideal; however, it may be unrealistic to achieve in all cases.

- *Loose/lenient criteria*. This requires no symptoms, no clinical signs of disease, and a decrease (or at least no increase) in the size of the preoperative periapical radiolucency for endodontic treatment to be deemed a success (Fig. 8.2a,b). This is a more realistic approach, especially as it is currently not possible to sterilize the entire root canal system so that it is microbe-free.

In the last decade a more pragmatic approach to categorizing the outcome of endodontic treatment has been suggested by assessing the survival of an endodontically treated tooth. This is defined as the patient being asymptomatic and able to use the endodontically treated tooth (known as an 'asymptomatic functional tooth'), this is similar to the criteria used to assess dental implants. It does not take into account whether periapical periodontitis has been cured or prevented following endodontic treatment. These new criteria are useful for comparing the outcome of endodontic treatment and the outcome of dental implant treatment.

Patients cannot make an informed decision on which treatment option to embark upon unless they are given knowledge of the expected treatment outcome, and how this compares to the outcome of other treatment options (e.g. implant retained crown or a bridge). It is also important for the clinician to explain this to patients from the outset.

The outcome of endodontic treatment is commonly categorized into either being a 'success' or 'failure'. These are subjective terms and one person may define success/failure completely differently from another person. Take, for example, an endodontically treated tooth which is symptom-free and functional; however, there is an associated sinus tract and periapical radiolucency which is increasing in size. A patient may perceive the endodontic treatment to have been a 'success' as they are not experiencing symptoms and can use their tooth. The patient may not even realize that there is a sinus tract present. From a clinician's point of view, this endodontic treatment has clearly not been a 'success'. The clinician may then inform the patient that the endodontic treatment has 'failed'. The patient may interpret this to mean the

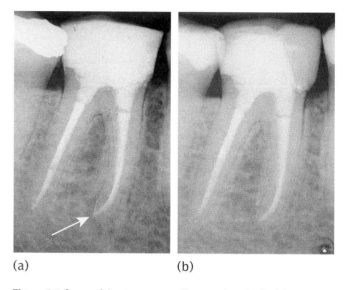

(a)   (b)

Figure 8.1 Successful outcome according to strict criteria: (a) immediate post-operative radiograph showing a periapical radiolucency (arrow); (b) radiograph taken one year later showing full resolution of the periapical radiolucency.

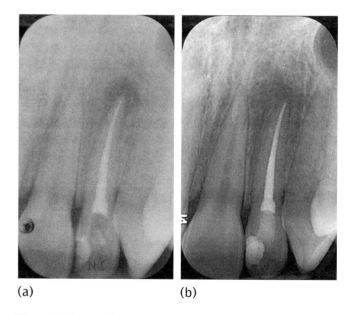

(a)   (b)

Figure 8.2 Successful outcome according to loose criteria: (a) immediate post-operative radiograph; (b) radiograph taken one year later showing a reduction in size of the periapical radiolucency. The patient was symptom-free. According to strict criteria, this case would not be considered a 'success' as there has not be full resolution of the periapical radiolucency.

clinician has failed in their abilities to carry out the procedure rather than there being persistent disease. For this reason, the authors suggest that the terms 'success' and 'failure' are avoided, or at least that the clinician define clearly their meanings to the patient in relation to the aim of endodontic treatment. Many other terms have been suggested for categorizing the outcome of endodontic treatment, e.g. 'healed/ healing/diseased' or 'effective/ineffective'. To comply with the current guidelines published by the European Society of Endodontology, the terms 'favourable', 'uncertain', and 'unfavourable' are used to categorize the outcome of endodontic treatment in this book.

What factors influence the outcome of root canal treatment and retreatment?

The outcome of root canal treatment and retreatment is very favourable; the probability of achieving a favourable outcome can be as high as 95 per cent. There are several prognostic factors which may influence the outcome of treatment (Table 8.1). The literature is replete with studies that have assessed the influence of these factors on the outcome of root canal treatment and retreatment. Systematic reviews have found it difficult to compare the results of all of these studies as there is so much variation in treatment protocols and the detail of the recorded data. Despite this heterogeneity, there is good evidence to support that three main prognostic factors influence the outcome of root canal treatment and retreatment, these are: the preoperative status of the periapical tissues, the quality and length of the root canal filling, and the quality of the coronal restoration.

Preoperative status of the periapical tissues

The outcome of endodontic treatment is more likely to be favourable in:

- Teeth with vital pulps (e.g. gross caries, elective endodontic treatment for post placement);
- Teeth with inflamed pulps (e.g. irreversible pulpitis);
- Teeth with necrotic uninfected pulps.

Radiographically, these teeth would not have signs of a preoperative periapical radiolucency. The probability of achieving a favourable outcome (i.e. maintaining a healthy periapical status) after endodontic treatment is in the region of 95 per cent.

In teeth with signs of periapical periodontitis (i.e. a periapical radiolucency on a radiograph) the probability of achieving a favourable outcome (i.e. curing an existing periapical periodontitis) after endodontic treatment is in the region of 85 per cent. This is likely to be due to teeth affected by periapical periodontitis having a more established infection in the root canal system when compared to teeth unaffected by periapical periodontitis.

The literature has conflicting conclusions on the influence of the size of the preoperative periapical lesion on outcome of treatment. The likelihood of a favourable outcome appears to be higher when the size of the preoperative periapical lesion is small (<5 mm).

Quality of the root canal filling

The outcome of endodontic treatment is more likely to be favourable when the quality of the root canal filling is satisfactory. A satisfactory root canal filling (as assessed radiographically) should extend to within 2 mm of the radiographic apex and should be well compacted. The radiographic quality of the root canal filling is an indicator of how well mechanical and chemical preparation of the root canal(s) were carried out to control infection, and also how well the root canal filling prevents reinfection. The likelihood of a favourable outcome is lower when:

- The root canal filling is overextended/'long' (Fig. 8.3a,b). This is essentially because microbes and infected debris are extruded into the periapical tissues. It is not necessarily due to the overextended root canal filling material itself.
- The root canal filling is underextended/'short' (Fig. 8.4a,b). This is because the portion of the root canal which does not contain any filling material is likely to contain residual microbes due to inadequate mechanical and chemical preparation.
- The root canal filling contains voids (Fig. 8.5a,b). This is because space(s) within the root canal filling may allow: (1) periapical tissue fluid to enter the root canal and provide a nutrient source of any residual microbes, (2) a place for any residual microbes to multiply, and (3) passage of microbes and their toxins from the root canal space into the periapical tissues.

Table 8.1 Factors that influence the outcome of root canal treatment and retreatment

Factors that influence outcome
- Preoperative status of the periapical tissues
- Quality of the root canal filling
- Quality of the coronal restoration

Factors that may influence outcome
- Medical status of the patient
- Preoperative sinus tract status
- Experience of the clinician
- Use of rubber dam
- Type of files used for preparation
- Type of irrigant used
- Number of visits to complete treatment
- Type of medicaments used
- Type of root canal filling used
- Technique used to fill the root canal

Factors that have no influence outcome
- Gender of patient
- Age of patient
- Type of tooth

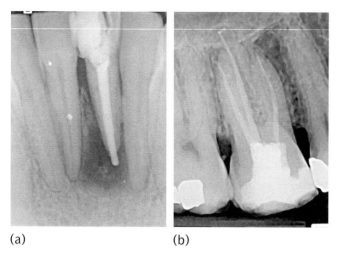

(a)   (b)

Figure 8.3 (a,b) Overextended root canal fillings and associated periapical radiolucencies.

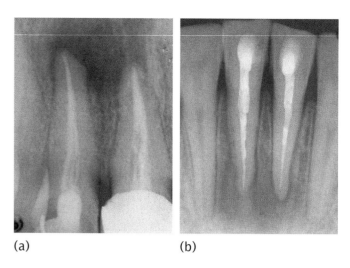

(a)   (b)

Figure 8.5 (a,b) Voids within root canal fillings and associated periapical radiolucencies.

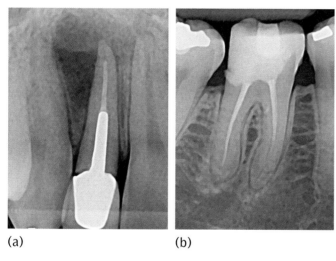

(a)   (b)

Figure 8.4 (a,b) Underextended root canal fillings with visible patent root canal space apically and associated periapical radiolucencies.

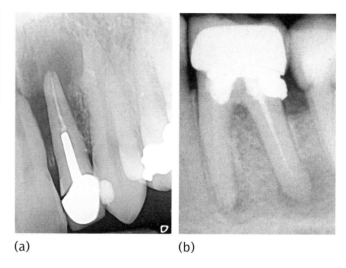

(a)   (b)

Figure 8.6 (a,b) Unsatisfactory quality root canal fillings and coronal restorations, and associated periapical radiolucencies.

In certain retreatment cases, it may not be possible to improve the quality of the existing root canal filling. This may be due to existing iatrogenic errors (e.g. ledges, transportation, perforations) that occurred during the primary root canal treatment. If the quality of the existing root canal filling cannot be improved and there are signs of periapical periodontitis, the outcome of root canal retreatment will be significantly reduced.

Quality of the coronal restoration

The outcome of endodontic treatment is more likely to be favourable when the quality of the coronal restoration is satisfactory. A satisfactory coronal restoration has no marginal deficiencies, defects, or recurrent caries. Deficiencies or defects associated with a coronal restoration present routes for reinfection of the root canal space from the mouth.

There has been much debate as to whether the quality of the root canal filling or the quality of the coronal restoration is more important. The probability of achieving a favourable outcome is reduced further when both the quality of the root canal filling and the quality of the coronal restoration are poor (Fig. 8.6a,b). It is recommended that both a satisfactory root canal filling and a satisfactory coronal restoration be provided to achieve a favourable outcome.

Other prognostic factors

Other factors may affect the outcome of endodontic treatment; however, there are either conflicting data or a paucity of evidence to confirm this. These include:

- *Medical status of the patient*. It has been suggested that the body's ability to heal periapical periodontitis may be impaired in certain medical conditions, e.g. patients with poorly controlled diabetes, patients on immunosuppressant medication.

- *Preoperative absence/presence of a sinus tract*. A sinus tract may indicate a higher number and/or virulence of endodontic microbes. There is some evidence to suggest that the probability of achieving a favourable outcome is higher with no preoperative sinus tract.

- *Experience of the clinician*, e.g. general dental practitioner versus a specialist in endodontics. There are no studies that compare directly the effect on outcome of the clinician's experience. The majority of cases in outcome studies are performed or supervised by endodontists. It could be argued from assessing the results of epidemiological studies that the probability of achieving a favourable outcome following endodontic treatment performed by a general dental practitioner will be slightly lower.

- *Use of rubber dam*. There is no strong evidence to suggest that the probability of achieving a favourable outcome will be higher with use of rubber dam. Ethically, it would not be possible to carry out a randomized controlled trial to test this. Despite the lack of evidence, there is a good clinical rationale for using rubber dam, in particular for infection control, and it remains a prerequisite for non-surgical endodontic treatment.

- *Type of files used for preparation*, e.g. stainless steel versus nickel-titanium (NiTi). There are many benefits to using NiTi file systems to prepare root canals (e.g. reduced mechanical preparation time, less clinician fatigue, reduced chance of iatrogenic errors); however, there is insufficient data to show that a particular type of file will achieve a higher outcome of endodontic treatment.

- *Type of irrigant used*. The probability of achieving a favourable outcome is, of course, higher with irrigants which are antimicrobial and can dissolve organic material. Sodium hypochlorite (NaOCl) is the gold standard irrigant and there is no strong evidence to suggest that any other irrigant on the market is superior.

- *Number of visits to complete treatment*. Traditionally, non-surgical endodontic treatment of teeth with infected necrotic root canal systems was carried out over multiple visits with an interappointment antimicrobial medicament. Newer research has challenged this and suggests that there is no significant difference in outcome between single and multiple visit treatment. There are many benefits to the clinician and patient in completing endodontic treatment in a single visit; however, this should not take precedence over planning or having sufficient time to thoroughly prepare the root canal system.

- *Type of interappointment medicament*. Many clinicians will have their personal preference for a particular type of medicament. There is no evidence to support that one type of medicament is more effective than another in terms of increasing the probability of achieving a favourable outcome.

- *Type of root canal filling material used*, e.g. gutta-percha (GP) versus polymer-based materials versus calcium silicate cements. In the 1990s there was a flurry of literature purporting that GP 'leaked', and polymer-based materials were more likely to seal the root canal system. The methodology and clinical relevance of these mainly laboratory-based studies has been criticized. Presently, there is insufficient data to suggest that one type of root canal filling material significantly increases the probability of achieving a favourable outcome.

- *Technique used to fill the root canal*, e.g. cold compaction versus warm compaction. There are many pros and cons to the various root canal filling techniques (see Chapter 6); however, there is no evidence to suggest that one technique increases the chance of a favourable outcome. The important factor is carrying out a satisfactory root canal filling.

There is no strong evidence to suggest that the following factors influence the outcome of endodontic treatment or retreatment:

- The gender of the patient;
- The age of the patient;
- Type of tooth, e.g. incisor versus molar.

What factors influence the outcome of surgical endodontics?

The probability of achieving a favourable outcome following surgical endodontics can be over 95 per cent (Fig. 8.7a,b). The outcome of surgical endodontics is more likely to be favourable when using:

- Contemporary surgical equipment (e.g. micro-surgical instruments, operating microscope/endoscope);

- Contemporary techniques (e.g. resecting the root-end without a bevel, using ultrasonics to prepare the root-end cavity);

- Contemporary materials (e.g. calcium silicate cements).

Foundations of clinical practice

The remainder of this chapter covers the practical aspects of assessing and classifying the outcome of endodontic treatment.

How do you assess the outcome of endodontic treatment?

Assessing the outcome of endodontic treatment is essentially assessing whether the aim of endodontic treatment has been fulfilled, i.e. to prevent or cure periapical periodontitis. The most accurate way to ensure there is no periapical periodontitis following endodontic treatment would be to carry out block dissection and serial histological sections of the tooth and surrounding jaw bone. Obviously this is extreme and not recommended! As clinicians, we instead rely on a clinical and radiographic review to assess outcome. A decision on the outcome of endodontic treatment can be reached once an objective comparison has been made between the findings of the preoperative/intraoperative and review appointments. The review appointment(s) should include:

- Assessment of the patient's symptoms;
- Clinical examination;
- Radiographic examination.

Endodontically treated teeth should be reviewed after treatment has been completed. Enough time should be given before arriving at a decision on the outcome of endodontic treatment—conventionally, this has been at least one year after treatment has been completed. A review at a few months after treatment is usually too early to definitively determine outcome. If patients are experiencing persistent or recurring symptoms, then review appointments should be scheduled as soon as

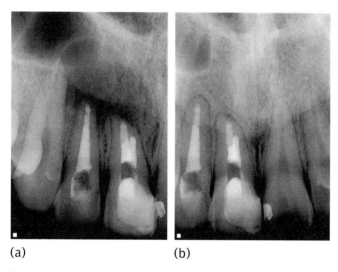

(a)   (b)

Figure 8.7 Radiographic evidence of a favourable outcome following surgical endodontics: (a) immediate post-operative radiograph; (b) radiograph taken one year later shows bony infill.

possible. Further review appointments may be necessary depending on if the outcome is deemed to be favourable, uncertain, or unfavourable (Fig. 8.8). Patients should be informed of the importance of review appointments from the outset.

Patients' symptoms

Sometimes patients may complain of pain, swelling, and/or loss of function at the review appointment. It is not wise to solely rely on patient symptoms to make a decision on the outcome of endodontic treatment. Care should be taken as symptoms can be subjective and the perception of pain can vary widely. Clinicians should avoid jumping to conclusions by assuming the endodontic treatment has 'failed' just because there are symptoms associated with an endodontically treated tooth. It is important to determine the cause(s) of the symptoms, in particular, is it odontogenic or non-odontogenic, and if odontogenic, is it endodontic or non-endodontic? For example, food trapping associated with a recently placed coronal restoration with poor contacts on an endodontically treated tooth may result in an inflamed gingival margin, the symptoms of which may mimic periapical periodontitis. If a patient is symptom-free at the review appointment, this does not necessarily represent a favourable outcome. It should be remembered that chronic periapical periodontitis is usually symptom-free. It is therefore important for the clinician to carry out an objective assessment, i.e. a clinical and radiographic examination.

Clinical examination

Illumination and, ideally, magnification are required when examining an endodontically treated tooth and the associated tissues. The following clinical findings should be assessed at the review appointment and then compared to the preoperative clinical findings:

- Presence/absence of a sinus tract or swelling in the associated soft tissues;
- Tenderness to palpation of the associated soft tissues;
- Tenderness to percussion of the endodontically treated tooth;
- Quality of the coronal restoration, e.g. deficient margins;

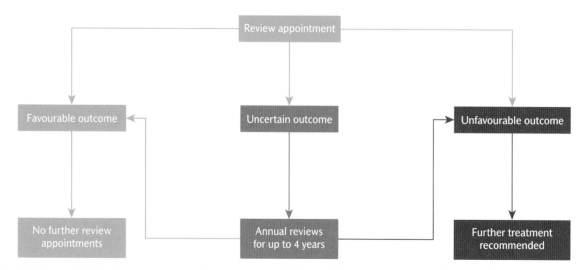

Figure 8.8 Diagram summarizing the review process (Adapted from guidelines published by the European Society of Endodontology).

- Presence of tooth fractures, including number, depth and extent;
- Presence of dental caries;
- Periodontal status: probing depths, mobility.

Radiographic examination

The endodontically treated tooth as a whole (not individual roots) should be assessed as the unit for outcome. To ensure a reliable comparison between preoperative/intraoperative and review radiographs, a paralleling technique, film holder, and aiming device should be utilized. Film-based radiographs should be viewed in optimal conditions, e.g. on a light box. Digital radiographic images should be adjusted to have suitable contrasts using computer software. The radiographic examination should include a report of:

- Quality of the root canal filling, i.e. extension ('length') and compaction (voids/no voids);
- Presence/absence of a periapical radiolucency;

- Size of the review periapical radiolucency, if present, and comparison of this to the size of the preoperative/intraoperative periapical status (increase, decrease, no change in size);
- Quality of the coronal restoration;
- Presence of dental caries;
- Periodontal status.

Conventional radiographs may be unable to detect periapical lesions due to superimposition of anatomical structures or geometric distortion. Cone beam computed tomography (CBCT) has a superior accuracy in detecting periapical lesions when compared to conventional radiographs. In certain cases, CBCT may be indicated to give a more objective and accurate determination of outcome of endodontic treatment (Fig. 8.9a,b,c,d). For example, CBCT may be indicated when a patient is complaining of symptoms but the conventional radiograph shows no periapical radiolucency. It would be recommended that these cases be referred to an endodontist for assessment.

How do you classify the outcome of endodontic treatment?

The outcome of endodontic treatment may be deemed to be favourable, uncertain, or unfavourable (see Table 8.2).

Criteria for a favourable outcome

For the outcome of endodontic treatment to be deemed favourable, the following criteria should be observed:

- The patient is symptom-free;
- The endodontically treated tooth is functional;
- Clinically, the associated tissues are healthy (Fig. 8.10a,b);
- Radiographically, the associated periapical tissues appear healthy (Fig. 8.1a,b) or there is evidence of healing by scar tissue formation.

Criteria for an uncertain outcome

In certain cases, the clinician may not be able to clearly classify the outcome of treatment as favourable or unfavourable:

- The patient may be complaining of symptoms or may be symptom-free;
- Clinically, there may be low-grade tenderness to palpation and/or percussion;
- Radiographically, the periapical radiolucency has persisted (remained the same size or only reduced in size) *within* the four-year assessment period (Fig. 8.11a,b).

Table 8.2 Classifying the outcome of endodontic treatment

	Favourable outcome	Uncertain outcome	Unfavourable outcome
Symptoms	No	Yes/No	Yes
Tooth functional	Yes	Yes/No	No
Clinical findings	Tooth and associated tissues appear healthy	Variable	Signs of infection, e.g. sinus tract, swelling, tenderness to palpation
Radiographic findings	Healthy periapical tissues	Same or reduced periapical radiolucency (within four years)	Increased periapical radiolucency Same or reduced periapical radiolucency (at or after four years)

Adapted from guidelines published by the European Society of Endodontology

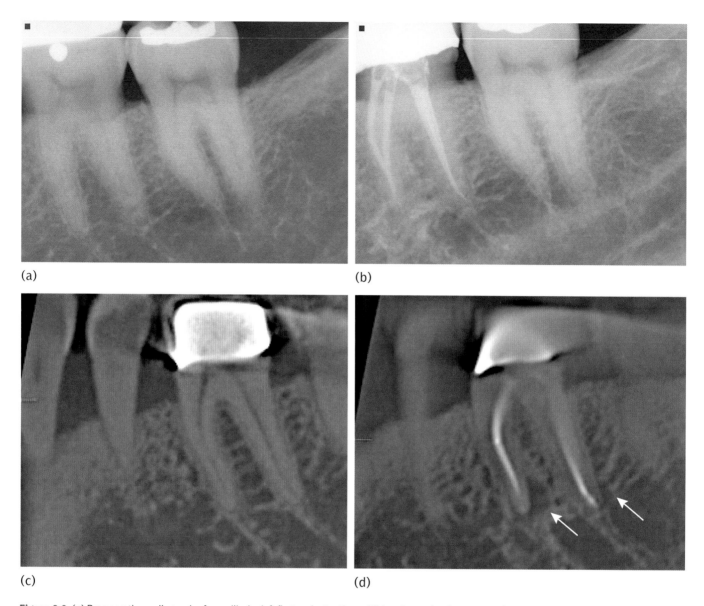

(a) (b)

(c) (d)

Figure 8.9 (a) Preoperative radiograph of mandibular left first molar tooth, and (b) radiograph taken 1 year after root canal treatment showing no periapical radiolucencies. (c-d) Reformatted cone beam computed tomography (CBCT) images reveal no preoperative periapical radiolucencies, but 1 year later, there are new periapical radiolucencies (as indicated by the arrows).

Adapted from Patel S, Wilson R, Dawood A, Foschi F, Mannocci F (2012) The detection of periapical pathosis using digital periapical radiography and cone beam computed tomography – Part 2: a 1-year post-treatment follow-up. *International Endodontic Journal* **45**, 711–23. Printed with permission from Wily-Blackwell.

Criteria for an unfavourable outcome

For the outcome of endodontic treatment to be deemed unfavourable, some of the following criteria may be observed:

- The patient is complaining of symptoms, e.g. pain, swelling;
- The endodontically treated tooth is not functional, e.g. the patient avoids eating on the tooth due to aggravation of symptoms;

- Clinically, there are signs of infection, e.g. sinus tract, swelling;
- Radiographically:
  — A new periapical radiolucency has developed post-treatment;
  — The periapical radiolucency has increased in size post-treatment (Fig. 8.12a,b).
  — The periapical radiolucency has persisted (remained the same size or only reduced in size) *at or after* a four-year assessment period.

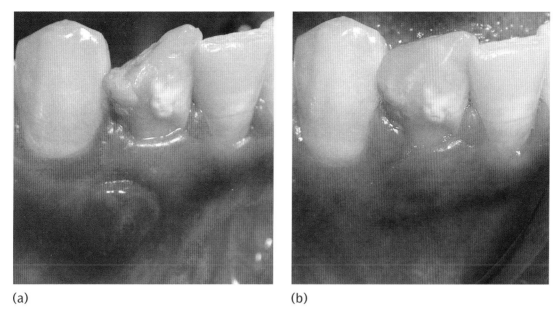

(a)   (b)

Figure 8.10 Clinical evidence of a favourable outcome associated with a mandibular lateral incisor tooth: (a) preoperative sinus tract; (b) the sinus tract has healed one year after endodontic treatment.

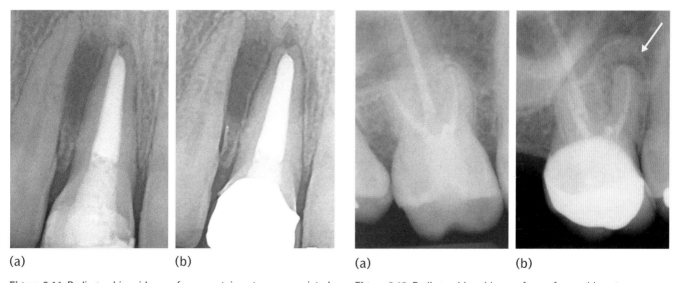

(a)   (b)   (a)   (b)

Figure 8.11 Radiographic evidence of an uncertain outcome associated with a maxillary central incisor tooth: (a) immediate post-operative radiograph; (b) radiograph taken one year later shows no change in the size of the periapical radiolucency.

Figure 8.12 Radiographic evidence of an unfavourable outcome associated with a maxillary first molar tooth: (a) immediate post-operative radiograph; (b) radiograph taken one year later shows an increase in the size of the periapical radiolucency (yellow arrow).

Conclusion

The key to achieving a favourable outcome after endodontic treatment is related to controlling infection of the root canal system (i.e. eliminating infection, and preventing reinfection). Clinicians should be striving to achieve higher treatment outcomes by taking a biological approach to endodontic treatment and not simply concentrating on achieving a radiopaque line in a root canal.

Summary points

- When assessing the outcome of endodontic treatment, we are essentially assessing whether we have been able to prevent or cure periapical periodontitis.

- Endodontically treated teeth should be reviewed to assess outcome—conventionally, this is done at least one year after the completion of endodontic treatment.

- The outcome of endodontic treatment may be deemed to be favourable, uncertain, or unfavourable. It is advisable to avoid using the terms 'success' and 'failure'.

- The probability of achieving a favourable outcome following endodontic treatment, i.e. the tooth is symptom-free and functional, and the associated tissues appear clinically and radiographically healthy, can be over 95 per cent.

- Three main prognostic factors influence the outcome of root canal treatment and retreatment: the preoperative status of the periapical tissues, the quality of the root canal filling, and the quality of the coronal restoration.

Suggested further reading

European Society of Endodontology (2006) Quality guidelines for endodontic treatment: consensus report of the European Society of Endodontology. *International Endodontic Journal* **39**, 921–30.

Figini L, Lodi G, Gorni F and Gagliani M (2007) Single versus multiple visits for endodontic treatment of permanent teeth. *Cochrane database of systematic reviews* **17**: CD005296.

Friedman S (2008) Expected outcomes in the prevention and treatment of apical periodontitis. In: Ørstavik D and Pitt Ford T (eds) *Essential endodontology: prevention and treatment of apical periodontitis*, 2nd edn; pp. 408–69. Oxford: Blackwell Munksgaard.

Ng YL, Mann V, Rahbaran S, Lewsey J and Gulabivala K (2008) Outcome of primary root canal treatment: systematic review of the literature—Part 2. Influence of clinical factors. *International Endodontic Journal* **41**, 6–31.

Torbinejad M, Lozada J, Puterman I and White SN (2008) Endodontic therapy or single tooth implant? A systematic review. *Journal of the California Dental Association* **36**: 429–37.

Online Resource Centre

To help you to develop and apply your knowledge and skills further, we have provided interactive learning resources online at http://www.oxfordtextbooks.co.uk/orc/patel/

9

Dealing with post-treatment disease

Shanon Patel and
Shalini Kanagasingam

Chapter contents

Introduction

This chapter will introduce the underlying theory of post-treatment disease before exploring how this transfers to clinical practice. It is important that you read the whole chapter to understand how theory and practice are related.

Understanding post-treatment disease

The outcome of endodontic treatment is influenced by biological and technical factors, including correct diagnosis, instrumentation, thorough disinfection, and root canal filling whilst respecting root canal morphology and avoiding complications during treatment. Despite endodontic treatment being one of the most technically demanding procedures in restorative dentistry, post-treatment disease is not very common. However, it is unwise to guarantee that endodontic treatment will be 100 per cent effective even if procedures have been performed with the greatest of care. Clinicians should always warn patients of the possible risks that accompany treatment, including post-treatment disease. It is important to understand the reasons for post-treatment disease so that it can be recognized and managed appropriately. Post-treatment disease should be looked upon as an opportunity for improvement and suitable steps should be taken to limit its recurrence.

The presence of microbes in the root canal system after endodontic treatment has been identified as the primary cause of post-treatment persistent (acute/chronic periapical periodontitis) disease (see Chapter 2). This is usually associated with inadequate root canal treatment, resulting in a persistent intraradicular infection. However, there are cases where the treatment has been carried out to the highest standards, yet post-treatment disease still occurs. This may be due to secondary intraradicular infection, i.e. the root canal has become reinfected (via the oral cavity) after the completion of root canal treatment. Apart from persistent and secondary intraradicular infection, extraradicular infections may also play a role in the failure of some cases. In addition, other non-microbial causes have also been implicated (Table 9.1).

How is post-treatment disease recognized?

The assessment of previous endodontic treatment should be based upon a sound history and symptoms reported by the patient, together with a thorough clinical and radiographic examination (see Chapters 3 and 8). When post-treatment disease is apparent, the cause needs to be established before deciding on the appropriate management. Post-treatment disease may be endodontic, periodontal, and/or prosthodontic in origin. The clinician should not automatically assume that the cause is endodontic in origin simply because a tooth has been endodontically treated.

Relevant history

Knowledge of the previous endodontic treatment is invaluable and every effort should be made to glean as much information as possible. This information may influence the possible treatments of the patient's specific endodontic problem. In addition to the routine questions asked during history taking, the following questions may be considered:

- *Where was the treatment performed?* The treatment may have been carried out in a dental hospital/University, general, or specialist practice. It is worthwhile establishing the name and whereabouts of the clinician as this will allow, when relevant, direct communication with the clinician who may offer more accurate details regarding the previous treatment.

Table 9.1 Causes of post-treatment endodontic disease

Intraradicular infection

- *Persistent infection*: Residual microbes left within the root canal system during previous endodontic treatment which survive and proliferate, especially in unfilled accessory and lateral canals.

- *Secondary infection*: Microbes may have re-entered the root canal system after completion of endodontic treatment. Routes of re-entry include fractures and coronal leakage (see Chapter 2).

Extraradicular infection

- Periapical actinomycosis, whereby actinomycotic bacteria form cohesive colonies, which enable them to escape the host defence system in the periapical tissues.

- Microbial infection of abscessed apical periodontitis lesions with or without sinus tracts.

- Infected root dentine debris displaced and inadvertently extruded into the periapical tissues during root canal instrumentation.

True cysts

- Apical true cysts are self-sustaining and independent of the presence or absence of root canal infection.

Foreign body reaction

- Foreign bodies such as gutta-percha (GP), paper points, and cholesterol crystals trapped in the periapical tissues during and after endodontic treatment can compromise healing.

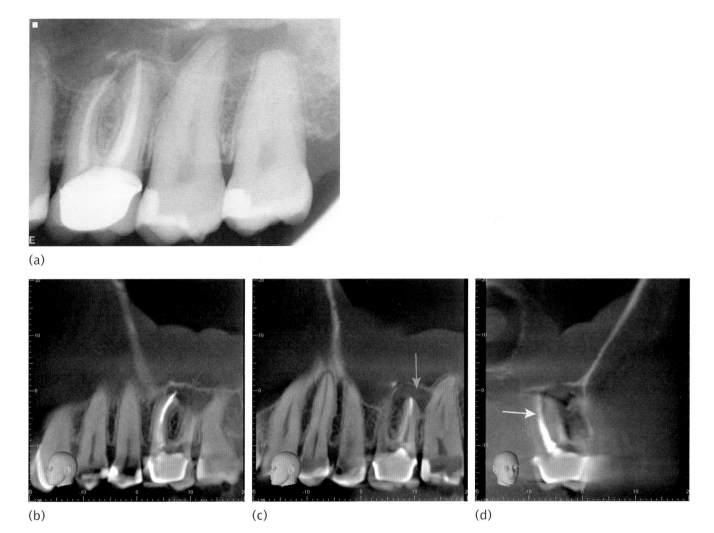

(a)

(b)   (c)   (d)

Figure 9.1 (a) Periapical radiograph of a symptomatic endodontically treated maxillary first molar tooth: the root canal fillings appear to be well compacted, but there has been an overextension associated with the mesio-buccal root. Reconstructed sagittal CBCT images reveal periapical radiolucencies associated with the (b) mesio-buccal root (red arrow) and (c) disto-buccal root (green arrow). (d) A reconstructed coronal CBCT image reveals voids within the palatal root canal filling (yellow arrow).

- *When was the treatment performed?* The timing of the previous endodontic treatment could help to differentiate between a healing versus a persisting periapical lesion. Endodontic treatment carried out recently could be associated with the former, whereas endodontic treatment carried out many years ago would most likely be associated with the latter.

- *What was the original diagnosis?* The patient may be able to provide information regarding the reason for the previous treatment. It may be possible to distinguish between a pulpal or periapical problem, and whether or not there was evidence of periapical radiolucency.

- *Was there any discomfort before, during, or immediately after treatment?* The patient may recall the timing, the nature of any pain experienced, and/or advice given by the clinician about the prognosis at the time of initial treatment. The likelihood of complications during treatment may be identified (e.g. separated instruments or perforations).

- *What techniques were used during the treatment?* Patients may remember the use of rubber dam and the taking of radiographs. They may not remember the names of irrigants or medicaments. They may, however, recall the odours (e.g. bleach) associated with their use. It should be possible to determine if the treatment was carried out in single or multiple appointments, including time devoted to each procedure.

The patient may also complain of typical signs of chronic periapical periodontitis, for example tenderness to chew or recurrent abscesses localized to the region of the previously root treated tooth. It is important to remember that the patient may be symptom-free, therefore, thorough clinical and radiographic examination is essential.

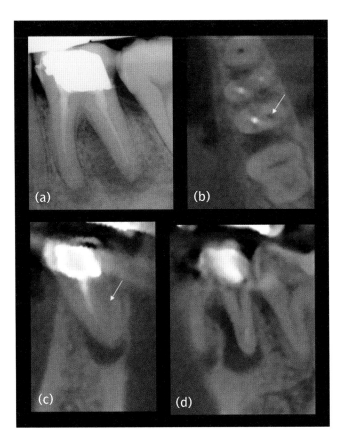

Figure 9.2 (a) Conventional radiograph of symptomatic mandibular molar. (b,c,d) Cone beam computed tomography (CBCT) reconstructed images of the same region: (b) axial and (c) coronal slices clearly show an unidentified disto-lingual root canal (arrows), (d) sagittal slice reveals the true extent of the bone loss around the distal root.

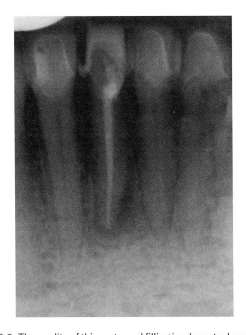

Figure 9.3 The quality of this root canal filling is adequate; however, a periapical radiolucency is still present after five years.

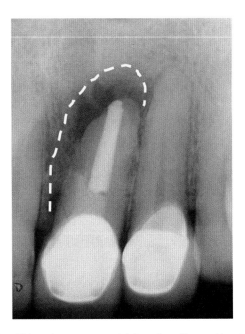

Figure 9.4 This patient was complaining of swelling and tenderness on biting associated with the maxillary central incisor tooth. A periapical radiograph revealed a J-shaped radiolucency (dashed line) which was due to a vertical root fracture.

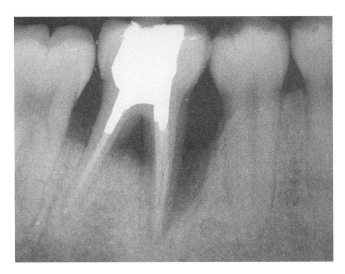

Figure 9.5 The quality of this root canal filling is adequate; however, the prognosis of the tooth is influenced by the extensive bone loss associated with the mesial root and the furcal region due to localized aggressive periodontitis.

Clinical and radiographic examination

Thorough extraoral and intraoral examination is essential to confirm the origin of post-treatment disease. As discussed previously (see Chapter 3 and 8), the absence of symptoms is not necessarily an indicator of the absence of disease. The clinical signs of tenderness to percussion or palpation and/or sinus tracts may indicate post-treatment disease. Radiographs are essential for detecting signs of periapical pathosis as well as evaluation of the quality of the existing root canal filling. Nonetheless, it must be noted that radiographs can only provide two-dimensional views of the area of interest (Fig. 9.1). CBCT scan may be helpful in confirming the presence of periapical lesions as well as the presence of unidentified root canals (Fig. 9.2). This information is essential to determine the cause, location and extent of the post-treatment disease.

Radiographs of endodontically treated teeth do not reveal a great deal about the biological status of the root canal system. An apparently well-filled root canal does not guarantee the absence of infection (Fig. 9.3). The root canal may in fact be heavily infected. When available, previous radiographs should be examined to identify possible changes in radiographic appearance of the periapical tissues; an increase in the size of a periapical radiolucency would indicate an unfavourable outcome.

Non-endodontic post-treatment disease

Alternative diagnoses should be considered for cases with post-treatment disease which have been carried out to a high standard, i.e. a good technical quality with strict adherence to aseptic treatment protocols (use of rubber dam, sodium hypochlorite). Some periapical radiolucencies may mimic clinical and radiographic features of periapical periodontitis. These dental problems include vertical root fracture and marginal periodontitis. Radiographically, an advanced case of vertical root fracture will exhibit a 'halo' or 'J-shaped' radiolucency, which differentiates it from the more spherical periapical radiolucency associated with persistent endodontic disease (Fig. 9.4). Teeth diagnosed with a vertical root fracture have a very poor prognosis and should ideally be extracted. The prognosis of an endodontically treated tooth with chronic periodontal disease will depend on the success of the periodontal therapy (Fig. 9.5).

What are the options for dealing with post-treatment disease?

There are several options available to manage post-treatment disease. These include:

- No treatment (keeping the tooth under review);
- Root canal retreatment;
- Surgical endodontics;
- Extraction.

The decision of which option to proceed with is based upon the strategic importance of the tooth, procedural complexities, clinician ability, patient preference, patient motivation, and costs. Complex procedures, such as root canal retreatment and surgical endodontics, are better dealt with by a specialist in endodontics and a referral should be offered to the patient.

No treatment (keeping the tooth under review)

There are cases where the outcome may not have been favourable according to strict criteria (i.e. complete resolution of a preoperative periapical radiolucency), but the tooth is stable enough to warrant review rather than intervention. This can often be the case in teeth that were endodontically treated many years previously and have remained symptom-free. Radiographic examination may reveal an existing periapical radiolucency which has stayed the same size since endodontic treatment was completed to a good standard (Fig. 9.6). In some cases a new periapical radiolucency will have emerged at the first review appointment; however, at subsequent review appointments the periapical radiolucency has stabilized and not increased in size.

Active treatment may carry certain risks and complications that are best avoided until there are symptoms (e.g. tenderness to chewing, acute pain) or signs (e.g. tenderness to buccal palpation, sinus tracts). An example of such a scenario might be a symptom-free endodontically treated tooth which has been restored with a well-fitting crown; however, a radiograph reveals a periapical radiolucency. In reality, this tooth is a candidate for root canal retreatment, however, treatment may be deferred if/when symptoms arise. The patient must be advised that they will require regular reviews to confirm that the existing radiolucency is not increasing in size, and that they should return if they develop any symptoms. The patient must also be warned of the possibility of an unexpected acute flare-up.

Root canal retreatment

Root canal retreatment is the treatment of choice when there is post-treatment endodontic disease associated with an inadequate root canal filling. Technically inadequate root canal fillings may indicate inadequate instrumentation and disinfection. Root canal retreatment should also be considered if there is evidence of coronal leakage. The goals of root canal retreatment are similar to those for root canal treatment; namely to eradicate microbes from the root canal system and provide a good apical and coronal seal to prevent reinfection. Re-entering the infected root canal system provides the best opportunity to eliminate microbes. When carried out to a high standard, the probability of achieving a favourable outcome following root canal retreatment can be higher than 90 per cent.

Prior to initiating retreatment, patients must be advised that :

- Root canal retreatment can only be carried out if the tooth is considered restorable. Initial investigation, including removal of the coronal restoration, may reveal underlying gross caries and/or catastrophic fractures rendering the tooth unrestorable.

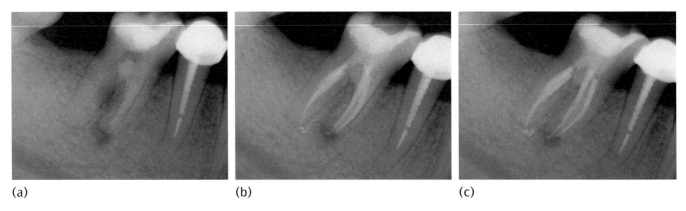

(a) (b) (c)

Figure 9.6 An endodontically treated mandibular molar that has remained symptom-free with a stable periapical radiolucency: (a) preoperative radiograph; (b) review radiograph at one year; (c) review radiograph at five years.

- Root canal retreatment is considered an advanced/complex procedure and there are potential risks involved in the removal of coronal restorations, root canal filling materials, posts, and separated instruments.

- The probability of a favourable outcome will be reduced if it is not possible to locate, fully instrument, and thoroughly disinfect the entire root canal system.

Management of existing extracoronal restorations

It is preferable to remove the entire crown to assess underlying tooth structure in order to confirm restorability of the tooth. Removal of the crown also improves access, which facilitates identification and improves access to all the root canals. In cases of old crowns or bridges, with marginal gaps, the choice is usually clear to dismantle them as part of the overall treatment plan. A satisfactory or recently placed crown or bridge may have to be removed if there is suspicion of secondary caries or a fracture. Once the extracoronal restoration is removed, a well-adapted provisional restoration may be placed to preserve structural integrity and prevent coronal leakage.

Occasionally, it may be possible to access through the crown or bridge (e.g. a recently placed crown); however, the patient must be advised that this restoration may have to be removed if there is difficulty locating and/or accessing all the root canals and/or caries is detected within the access cavity.

Removal of posts

Posts should be removed to allow access to the root canal for complete disinfection. The removal of posts can be a challenging and a potentially hazardous process as there is a risk of root fracture or propagation of microfracture lines. Cases should be assessed based on the following factors:

- Length and width of the post (longer and larger posts may be more difficult to remove);

- Post design (parallel, tapered, or threaded);

- Post material (metal posts are usually easier to remove compared to fibre posts);

- Type of cement (adhesive luting cements are more difficult to remove);

- History of decementation (a post-retained crown that has repeatedly decemented will be relatively easier to remove).

Some posts may be virtually impossible to remove (e.g. glass fibre posts cemented with adhesive cements) and/or may pose too high a risk for root fracture if removal was attempted (e.g. long, wide posts). These situations may warrant alternative treatment such as surgical endodontics. If it is possible to remove the coronal restoration and post, the tooth may be root canal treated or retreated (Fig. 9.7).

Removal of root canal filling materials

Gutta-percha (GP) is the most commonly used material for root canal filling. With the right technique, GP is relatively easy to remove from the root canal system. Other root canal filling materials may be challenging to remove:

- Carrier-based systems (e.g. Thermafil; Dentsply-Maillefer, Ballaigues, Switzerland).

- Hard-setting pastes and resins (e.g. resocrin-formaldehyde Russian Red (Fig. 9.8)).

- Silver points, especially those that are tightly wedged into the apical portion of the root canal.

It is essential to remove all of the existing root canal filling material. Remnants of materials are likely to harbour microbes which could compromise the disinfection process, and ultimately the outcome of retreatment. Retrieval of root canal filling materials often entails removal of dentine from around the coronal aspect of the root canal. Care should be taken to conserve as much sound tooth structure as possible.

Surgical endodontics

Surgical endodontics should only be considered when it is not possible (or pragmatic) to carry out root canal retreatment. The indications for surgery are limited to specific situations (Table 9.2). The biological rationale of surgical treatment remains similar to non-surgical treatment, namely the disinfection and sealing of the apical root canal system (Fig. 9.9).

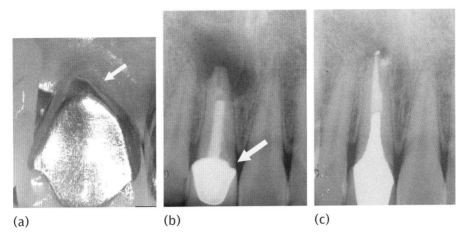

(a)   (b)   (c)

Figure 9.7 Endodontic treatment involving post removal: (a) the existing crown has deficient margins (yellow arrow); (b) preoperative radiograph showing deficient margin (yellow arrow) and large periapical radiolucency; (c) review radiograph showing a decrease in the size of the periapical radiolucency one year after root canal retreatment and a new post retained coronal restoration.

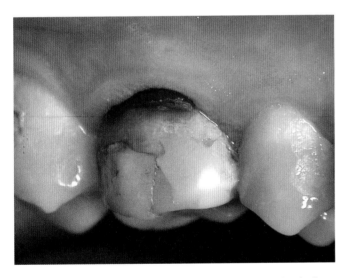

Figure 9.8 A maxillary first molar tooth that has been endodontically treated with 'Russian Red' resin.

Table 9.2 Indications and contraindications for surgical endodontics

Indications for surgical endodontics

- Root canal retreatment deemed to have an unfavourable outcome.
- Obstructions within the root canal (irretrievable separated instruments, calcified root canals, insoluble endodontic materials) which hinders instrumentation and disinfection.
- Teeth with long and wide diameter posts which pose a high risk of root fracture if retrieval was attempted via root canal retreatment.
- Perforations which require surgical repair.
- Investigative procedures (biopsies or confirmation of suspected vertical root fractures).
- Extraradicular infections and true cysts.

Contraindications to surgical endodontics

- Patient's medical history (e.g. bisphosphonates).
- Anatomical factors (e.g. sites which lack surgical access).
- Lack of expertise and equipment.

Root-end filling materials must be biocompatible, readily adapted to the root surface, and non-resorbable. The current materials of choice are zinc oxide-based materials, e.g. IRM (Dentsply, Tulsa, OK, USA), bioactive materials, e.g. ProRoot MTA (Dentsply, Tulsa, OK, USA), and there is emerging evidence for the use of Biodentine (Septodont, Saint Maur des Fossés, France).

The prognosis of endodontic surgery relies on meticulous patient assessment, diagnosis, and appropriate treatment planning. Traditional radiographic techniques, as well as newer imaging techniques such as CBCT, provide the clinician with the necessary information for optimal assessment of the surgical site. The advent of micro-surgical techniques and the development of new root-end filling materials have directly contributed to a high probability of a favourable outcome.

Extraction

There are situations where extraction may be in the patient's best interest. Extraction remains the most expedient method of treating endodontic disease. With extraction of the tooth, the microbes are eradicated and no longer have an effect on the host defence mechanisms. Indications for extraction are:

- Teeth which are considered to have questionable restorability;
- Non-functional teeth;

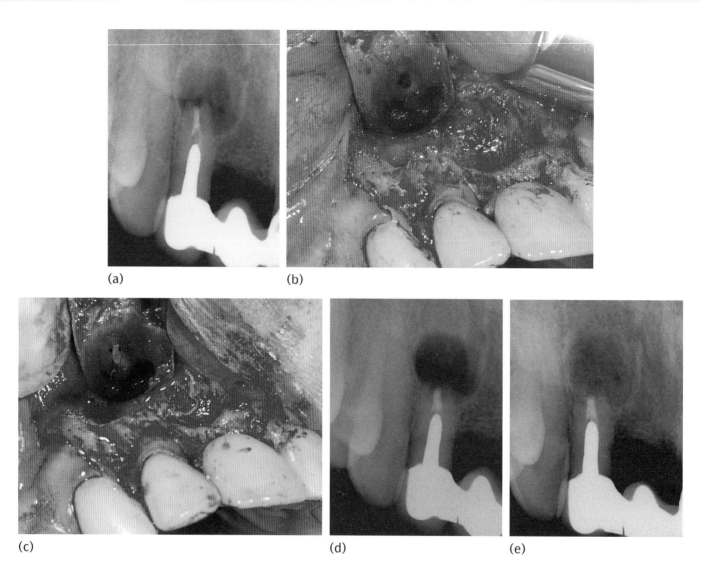

(a)   (b)

(c)   (d)   (e)

Figure 9.9 Surgical endodontics: the patient did not want to proceed with root canal retreatment due to the risk of root fracture during post removal and loss of the existing well-fitting bridge. (a) Preoperative radiograph showing wide post, unsatisfactory root canal filling, and a periapical radiolucency; (b) view of the root-end cavity following preparation using ultrasonics; (c) view of the new root-end filling; (d) immediate post-operative radiograph showing compacted root-end filling; (e) radiograph taken one year later showing significant bony infill.

- Teeth with no strategic value;
- Teeth with untreatable disease: vertical root fracture (Fig. 9.4), severe marginal periodontitis (Fig. 9.5), or gross caries.

If extraction is the treatment of choice, then the clinician should advise the patient on the various replacement options, including an implant-retained crown or a bridge.

Referring patients

One of the most difficult situations to deal with is the failure to appreciate when one's own clinical experience and ability is insufficient to deal with the needs and demands of a patient. When the patient's expectations are beyond the comfort zone of the clinician, a referral must be considered. Referral may be based not just on technical considerations but may be related to general patient management. Ideally, it is better to identify potential difficulties before commencing treatment so that the patient can be referred to a more experienced colleague, who can then manage the endodontic problem more appropriately. Complex procedures such as root canal retreatment and surgical endodontics are better dealt with by a specialist in endodontics.

Referral may be required after treatment has been initiated, and when clinical situations become unmanageable. These include irresolvable pain, acute exacerbations, procedural accidents (for example, separated instruments and perforations), or the inability to locate root canals.

Communication with the patient and the specialist in endodontics should be conducted in a manner that prevents any misunderstanding. A detailed letter explaining the situation and details of any treatment performed along with accompanying radiographs should be forwarded to the specialist in endodontics.

Foundations of clinical practice

The remainder of this chapter is concerned with the practicalities of dealing with post-treatment disease. The first section describes different techniques to aid the dismantling of crowns and bridges, after which techniques to remove the existing root canal filling materials are discussed. This chapter concludes with a discussion of the principles of surgical endodontics. It must be emphasized that these are advanced procedures and consideration should be given to referral to specialist in endodontics.

How are crowns/bridges removed?

Satisfactory coronal restorations can be preserved as long as they do not compromise access to the root canal system. Most cases would benefit from removal of the existing crowns or bridges as this would confirm the restorability of the tooth as well as improve access for retrieval of the existing root canal filling materials.

A variety of devices are available to remove single or multiple unit prostheses. One such device is the crown and bridge remover, which should be used with care (Fig. 9.10). Tapping crowns and bridgework off with such instruments may lead to fracture of the tooth.

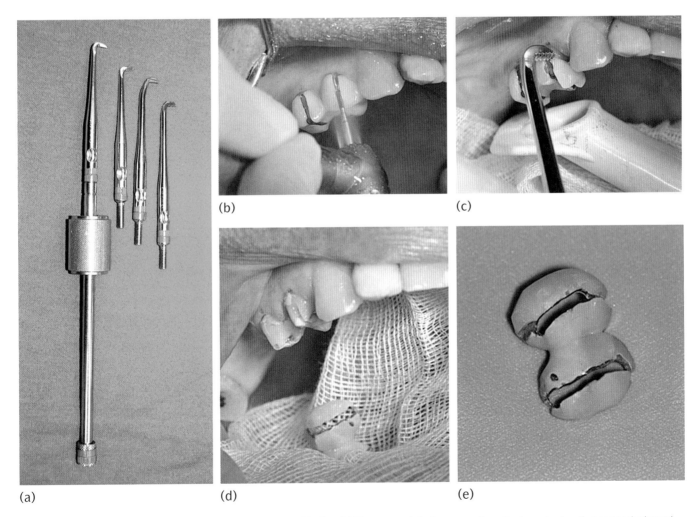

(a) (b) (c) (d) (e)

Figure 9.10 (a) A crown and bridge remover with interchangeable tips. (b) Slots are cut into the crowns from the buccal extending across the buccal surface. (c) The tip of the device is placed over the margin of the crown and tooth. The crown is then gently tapped away from the tooth. (d) The crowns are dislodged and caught in the protective gauze. (e) The retrieved crowns.

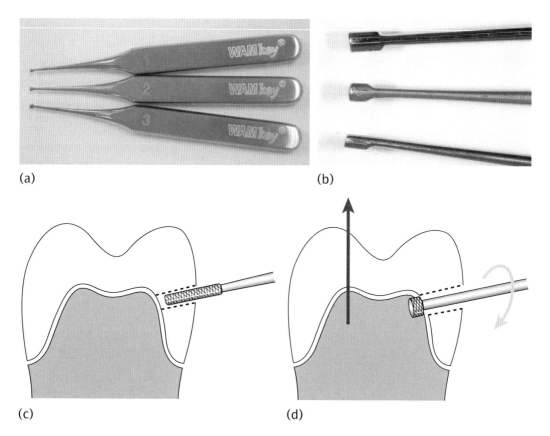

Figure 9.11 (a) WAMkeys (WAM, Aix-en Provence, France) with 3 different tips. (b) WAMkey tips enlarged. (c) A window is cut through the crown with a bur between the fitting surface of the crown and the occlusal surface of the prepared tooth structure. (d) A dissociating force (arrows) is applied with the WAMkey to remove the crown.

The WAMkey (WAM, Aix-en Provence, France) is an alternative device for removing crowns and bridges. First, a window is cut through the crown, and this device is then used to apply a dissociating force between the preparation's occlusal surface and the fit surface of the occlusal aspect of the crown (Fig. 9.11). This results in the removal of the intact crown, which can then be reused provisionally (Fig. 9.12) or in some cases (where the crown margins have not been altered), permanently recemented after retreatment.

Fixed restorations that are very retentive, or have been cemented with adhesive cements, are likely to require removal by sectioning. Burs should be chosen according to the crown material; porcelain can be sectioned with diamond burs, whereas metal removal is achieved more efficiently using tungsten carbide burs. Care must be taken to minimize the removal of the underlying sound tooth structure whilst removing the crowns and bridges.

How are core filling materials removed?

The most commonly used core filling materials are amalgam and composite resin. The bulk of material may be carefully cut away with long shank burs to improve visibility. The use of ultrasonic tips, under magnification, is ideal for removal of the remainder of material lying close to dentine. These tips are designed to remove controlled amounts of material, therefore preserving sound dentine.

Prolonged, continuous usage of ultrasonic tips should be avoided as this may cause overheating of the tooth and periapical tissues. This can be prevented by using water irrigation. Care should be taken to preserve the coronal portions of materials such as posts, silver points, and Thermafil carriers in order to facilitate their retrieval at a later stage.

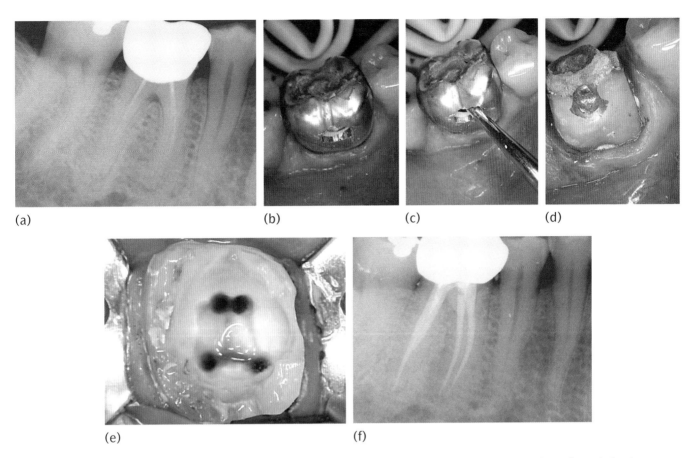

(a)　　　　　(b)　　　　　(c)　　　　　(d)

(e)　　　　　(f)

Figure 9.12 Root canal retreatment of a mandibular first molar tooth involving crown removal and reuse: (a) preoperative radiograph showing unsatisfactory root canal filling and periapical radiolucencies; (b) a window has been cut through the buccal surface of the crown; (c,d) crown is removed; (e) appearance of disinfected and prepared root canals; (f) immediate post-operative radiograph showing satisfactory root canal filling. The existing crown has been recemented as a provisional restoration.

How are posts removed?

Most posts can be dislodged using ultrasonic vibration to disturb the cement securing the post into the root canal, transmitted via specifically designed endodontic ultrasonic tips (Fig. 9.13). A forcep-type instrument, e.g. Steiglitz forceps (Hu-Friedy, Rotterdam, Netherlands), may then be used to retrieve the post (Fig. 9.14).

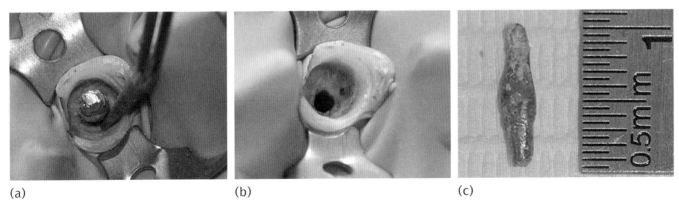

(a)　　　　　(b)　　　　　(c)

Figure 9.13 Metal post removal: (a) an ultrasonic tip is moved around the coronal portion of the post, transferring energy to break the cement bond; (b,c) post has been removed.

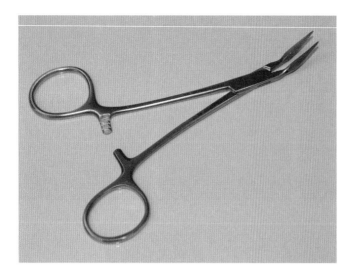

Figure 9.14 Steiglitz forceps (Hu-Friedy, Rotterdam, Netherlands).

If the post has not loosened after using ultrasonics, consideration can be given to a range of post-pulling devices. These include the Eggler post remover (Automaton-Vertriebs-Gesellschaft, Stuttgart, Germany), Thomas Universal Post Remover (FFDM-PNEUMAT, Bourges, France), and Ruddle post removal system (SybronEndo, Orange, CA, USA) (Fig. 9.15). There is the risk of root fracture if these devices are not used with care. Alternatively, the post may be drilled out piece by piece using a long shank bur. This should only be attempted by a competent clinician utilising magnification and coaxial illumination.

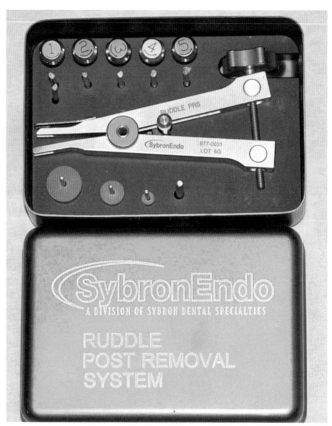

Figure 9.15 Ruddle post removal system (SybronEndo, Orange, CA, USA).

How are root canal filling materials removed?

There are various techniques which can be employed to remove root canal filling materials depending on the type of material (Table 9.3).

Gutta-percha can usually be retrieved manually using Hedström files (Fig. 9.16), alternatively, other techniques may be used (Table 9.3). There are several kits available which are specifically designed to remove silver points and separated instruments from the root canal system. The Masserann kit (Micro-Mega, Besancon, France) (Fig. 9.17) consists of

trepan burs and extractor devices. The trepan burs are selected to have slightly larger internal diameter than the obstruction and they are used to trough around the obstruction to facilitate its removal. The extractor is essentially a rod that is screwed into a tube. The tube is placed over the fragment to be removed and the rod is screwed home to grip it. The device can result in excessive removal of sound dentine thus weakening the tooth further.

Surgical endodontics

The scope of the surgical endodontics includes: incisional drainage and trephination, apical surgery, root resection, tooth resection, replantation, and biopsy.

Incisional drainage and trephination

The incision of a fluctuant swelling to drain pus can result in immediate pain relief and bring spreading infection under control. In the absence of a fluctuant swelling, where infection is confined to cancellous bone, the process of trephination may be employed. This involves drilling through the cortical bone to effect drainage. Trephination can lead to damage of adjacent dental structures and should only be carried out by a competent clinician.

Apical surgery

This involves apical curettage, root-end resection, root-end preparation, and root-end filling. Apical surgery requires special instruments and equipment (Fig. 9.18a).

Tissue flap reflection to provide vision and access is a fundamental consideration. There are many full and limited flap designs described according to their shapes and position. Flaps should consist of the full thickness of periosteum, mucosa, and gingival tissues. Flap reflection should be performed using appropriate elevators commencing away from the gingival margin. The flap should be lifted cleanly, separating the periosteum from the underlying

Table 9.3 Techniques for removal of root canal filling materials

Material	Removal technique
Gutta-percha (GP)	• Hedström file technique A Hedström file may be used to grasp and remove GP. This is especially effective in cases where single GP points have been used to fill the root canal (Figure 9.16). • Gates Glidden drill and rotary nickel-titanium (NiTi) technique Using a 'crown-down' approach, Gates Glidden drills are used to flare and remove GP from the coronal portion of the root canal. Rotary NiTi files can then be used to remove GP from the apical portion of the root canal. • Retreatment rotary NiTi technique Specially-designed files (e.g. ProTaper Universal Retreatment files; Dentsply Maillefer, Ballaigues, Switzerland) aid removal of the bulk of GP. As the file lengths are limited, the apical portion of the root canal may require hand instrumentation. • Solvent technique A solvent (e.g. chloroform) softens and dissolves GP and sealers. It is advisable to use solvents sparingly in order to avoid smearing GP along the root canal walls, which will be difficult to fully remove.
Paste	• Set pastes can be removed with ultrasonics and solvents. • Softened pastes can be removed by rotary NiTi or hand-files.
Plastic Core Carriers	• Ultrasonic tips can be used to free the plastic core carriers from surrounding materials. Then, the following techniques may be used: — Steiglitz forceps (Hu-Friedy, Rotterdam, Netherlands) can be used to grasp the plastic core to remove it. — Hedström file technique with or without solvent. — Braiding 2–3 Hedström files around the core. Retrieval of the files (engaged to the core) with a surgical needle holder levering against a cusp.
Silver points	• By creating a trough around the silver point (with ultrasonics), Steiglitz forceps can be used to grasp and remove the silver point. • Hedström-file braiding technique, withdrawn simultaneously.

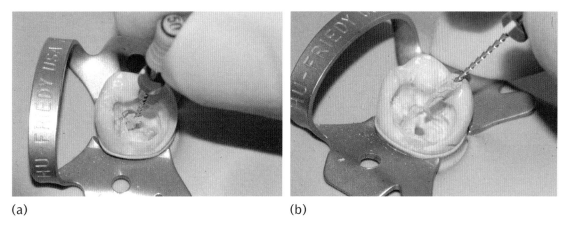

(a) (b)

Figure 9.16 A Hedström file has been used to grasp and remove GP.

bone. Once reflected, the tissue is held away from the surgical site by placing the retractor on bone to avoid tissue pinching. Regular irrigation of the surgical site prevents dehydration of the tissues. Location and identification of the root apex can be achieved using preoperative radiographs (including a CBCT scan), magnification, the presence of fenestration of the overlying cortical bone, and a sharp, straight probe.

Apical curettage involves the removal of a soft tissue lesion from around the root tip, before or after root-end resection perpendicular to the long axis of the root. A root-end cavity is prepared using ultrasonic retrotips (Fig. 9.18b) and then sealed to prevent the egress of residual microbes and their products. Bioactive materials such as calcium silicate materials are the recommended material for this purpose.

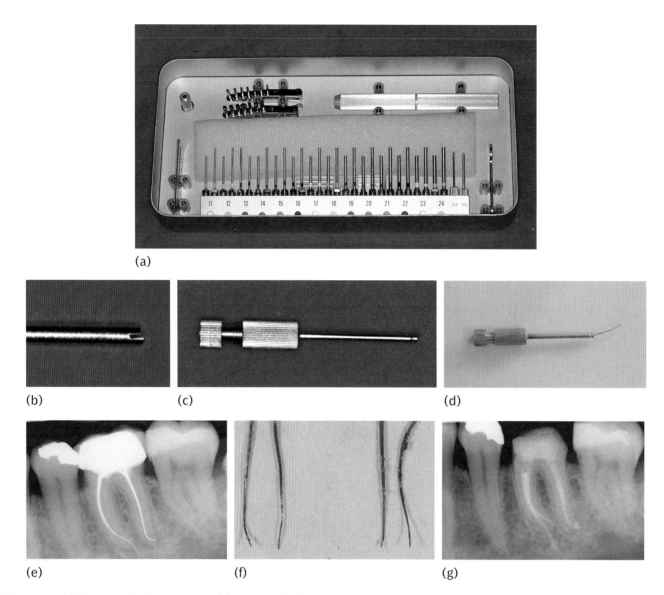

Figure 9.17 (a) Masserann kit; (b) a trepan bur; (c) extractor; (d) silver point retrieved using the Masserann kit (Micro-Mega, Besancon, France) ; (e) persistent disease associated with a mandibular molar tooth which has been root canal filled with silver points; (f) silver points retrieved using Masserann kit; (g) root canal retreatment carried and root canals filled with GP.

Wound closure involves the placement of sutures. The sutured flap should be held under gentle pressure for 5–10 min before discharging the patient with appropriate post-operative instructions. Sutures can be removed in 3–5 days. Residual scarring may arise in areas of sinus tract healing, relieving incisions, and suture placement where surgical technique has been poor.

Cases that require endodontic surgery should be referred to a specialist in endodontics.

The following sections are provided for further information only. There is no suggestion that the undergraduate dental student or recent graduate would perform these techniques. It is important, however, that you gain a working knowledge of the processes involved and cases that may be indicated for such treatment measures.

Corrective surgery

Corrective surgery is often performed to repair perforation defects in the root surface created iatrogenically. Calcium silicate cements are the materials of choice for this purpose.

Root resection

Root resection is the complete removal of a root from a multi-rooted tooth without interfering with the crown (Fig. 9.19). The indications for this procedure are severe periodontal disease, resorption, and vertical fractures. The procedure usually involves flap reflection, bone remodelling, and crown contouring to assist with plaque control.

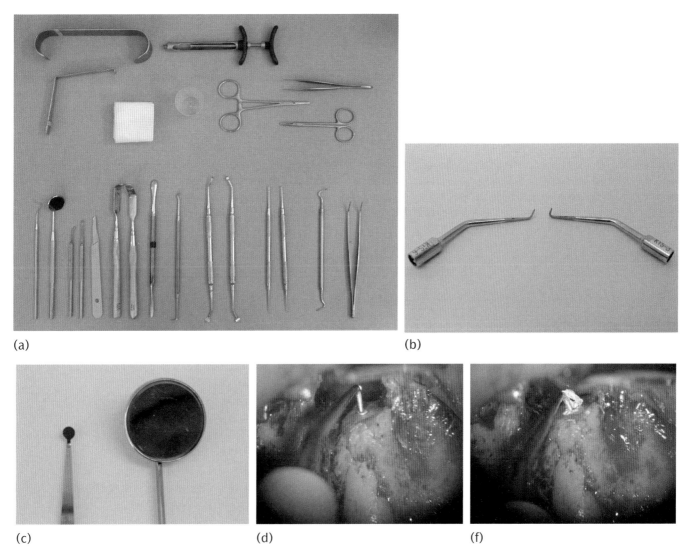

(a)

(b)

(c)

(d)

(f)

Figure 9.18 (a) Endodontic micro-surgery kit; (b) surgical ultrasonic retrotips allow improved access for minimal preparation of the apical portion of the root canal; (c) a surgical micromirror compared to a conventional mouth mirror; (d) and (e) surgical ultrasonic retrotip used to prepare a root-end cavity.

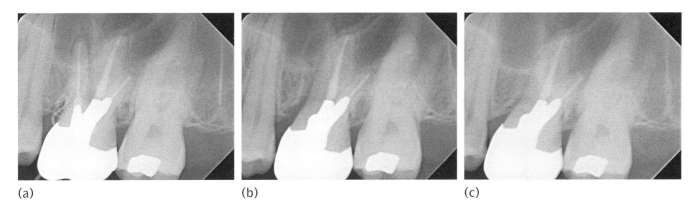

(a)

(b)

(c)

Figure 9.19 Root resection: (a) radiograph showing persistent disease, a GP point has been used to track a sinus adjacent to the mesio-buccal root; (b) radiograph showing root resection of the mesio-buccal root; (c) review radiograph taken 15 years later. Courtesy of Dr Tom Bereznicki.

Tooth resection

Tooth resection is slightly different from root resection in that it involves the cutting off of associated crown material along with root. A portion of the tooth is usually extracted and the remaining part is restored. Occasionally, both parts are retained and restored in a process often referred to as bicuspidization.

Replantation

Replantation may be performed intentionally in situations where other surgical options are not indicated. In essence, the tooth is extracted and modified out of the mouth in such a way as to facilitate the disinfection and sealing of the root canals. The tooth is returned to its socket and splinted for less than a week. An example would be a mandibular premolar, which was extracted and replanted to avoid apical surgery and the potential risk of damage to the mental nerve.

Marsupialization and decompression

Large periapical lesions may be treated by a surgical technique that involves penetration of the lesion through the cortical plate. Patency of the fistula is maintained by the use of a drain or, preferably, a flanged cannula. The marsupialized lesion may be irrigated and, with time, the lesion reduces in size until the decompression can be terminated.

Biopsy

Any tissue removed during surgery *must* be sent for routine histological examination to confirm the nature of the lesion. The sample should be forwarded for examination in 10 per cent formalin and should be accompanied with comprehensive case details.

Summary points

- It is important to recognize post-treatment disease and to identify the potential causes of persistent disease in order to formulate a comprehensive treatment plan.
- Persistent infection of the root canal is usually associated with poor technical quality of endodontic treatment. However, even well-treated teeth may harbour microbes which may prevent healing.
- Non-surgical root canal retreatment should always be considered as the first line of treatment if endodontic intervention is required.
- Alternative causative factors should be considered in cases which are resistant to root canal retreatment. These may include the presence of extraradicular infection and vertical root fracture.
- The restorability of a tooth must be confirmed prior to embarking on complex retreatment procedures.
- The outcome of root canal retreatment will depend on the removal the previous root canal filling material, full negotiation, and thorough disinfection of the entire root canal system.
- Surgical endodontics is indicated if root canal retreatment has not achieved a favourable outcome or is impracticable.

 Suggested further reading

Chong BS, Pitt Ford TR and Hudson MB (2003) A prospective clinical study of Mineral Trioxide Aggregate and IRM when used as root-end filling materials in endodontic surgery. *International Endodontic Journal* **36**, 520–6.

Gorni FG and Gagliani MM (2004) The outcome of endodontic retreatment: a 2 year follow-up. *Journal of Endodontics* **30**, 1–4.

Kim S and Kratchman S (2006) Modern endodontic surgery concepts and practice: a review. *Journal of Endodontics* **32**, 601–23.

Nair PNR (2004) Pathogenesis of apical periodontitis and the causes of endodontic failures. *Critical reviews in Oral Biology and Medicine* **15**, 348–81.

Torabinejad M, Corr R, Handysides R and Shabahang S (2009) Outcomes of non-surgical retreatment and endodontic surgery: a systematic review. *Journal of Endodontics* **35**, 930–7.

Online Resource Centre

 To help you to develop and apply your knowledge and skills further, we have provided interactive learning resources online at http://www.oxfordtextbooks.co.uk/orc/patel/

10

Dento-legal aspects of endodontics

Len D'Cruz

Chapter contents

Introduction

With modern techniques and materials, root canal treatment is being undertaken more often by dentists and more predictable results are being achieved. Patients are increasingly keener to retain their teeth, and their expectations of success are higher than they have been in the past. The standards expected of dentists in delivering care has been driven by regulatory bodies, litigation, and specialist societies. In primary dental care in the UK, endodontics has the highest number of legal claims in comparison with other dental treatments (Table. 10.1).

There are a range of complaints and claims that may arise in relation to endodontics (Fig. 10.1). Many complaints and clinical negligence claims arise out of the clinician's failure to communicate well with the patient. Even when something does go wrong, research has shown that explanations, empathy, and openness with the patient prevents an escalation of the problem. This chapter aims to discuss these dento-legal issues and the factors involved in reducing and managing risk in endodontics.

What is consent?

Consent is not a single event but a process. A good working definition from the Department of Health in England is:

> The voluntary, continuing permission of the patient to receive particular treatments. It must be based upon the patient's adequate knowledge of the *purpose, nature, likely effects,* and *risks* of that treatment including the likelihood of its *success* and a discussion of any alternative to it including no treatment.

There are some key elements in this definition which have been set out in italic and each time root canal treatment is contemplated, it is incumbent on the clinician to provide the information with specific reference to the patient and their tooth.

The significance of 'continuing permission' is very important. Take, for example, a patient who is undergoing root canal treatment on a molar tooth. If, during the procedure a difficulty is encountered, such as a curved or calcified root canal, further consent is required if the outcome of the treatment may be compromised (e.g. the inability to prepare the entire root canal to the desired length) and the prevailing situation is different from when treatment commenced. This further consent procedure enables the patient to weigh up the risks of continuing (or leaving part of the root canal unprepared and unfilled) against a decision to extract the tooth or accept a referral to a specialist in endodontics.

There are three essential and interdependent components to valid consent:

- *Competence*. The patient has sufficient ability to understand the nature of the treatment and the consequences of receiving or declining that treatment. The legal term is 'capacity'.
- *Voluntariness*. The patients has fully agreed to have the treatment and there has been no coercion or undue influence to accept or decline the treatment.
- *Information and knowledge*. The patient has been given sufficient and comprehensible information regarding the nature and consequences of the proposed and alternative treatments.

How much information should be given to a patient about endodontic treatment?

The simple answer is whatever is normal practice for a dentist to advise their patient. This is the professional test and was set out in

Table 10.1 Number of claims in primary dental care in UK

1) Endodontics
2) Crown and bridgework
3) Nerve damage
4) Oral surgery (except 3,7,10)
5) Periodontics
6) Orthodontics
7) Implants
8) Veneers
9) Dentures
10) Failure to diagnose/ treat

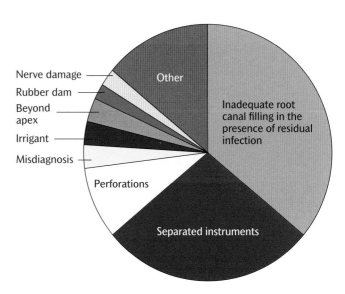

Figure 10.1 Range of complaints and claims in relation to endodontics in 2011 in the UK.

the case of Sidaway, the leading case in English law of this nature, and uses the 'Bolam test' as its basis. In other words, if it is not generally appropriate to warn about something, a dentist cannot be found guilty of negligence if they fail to warn. This is, however, modified by two important considerations. The first relates to the case of Bolitho where there were conflicting views about a clinical intervention. The House of Lords decided that whilst an opinion may be responsible, reasonable, and respectable, if it did not stand up to logic then it should not be accepted. The second consideration is the concept not of what a reasonable dentist may wish to advise a patient about a particular treatment, but what a reasonable patient might wish to hear. This is known as the 'prudent patient' test or objective test. This is a very patient-centred approach and creates a significantly higher burden on the dentist to provide appropriate information with which the patient can make decisions. This means that giving the 'usual warnings' about a particular procedure may not be sufficient if a patient is likely to attach more significance to one particular risk than another.

Endodontic treatment can be time-consuming and expensive (e.g. using nickel-titanium (NiTi) files). Whilst in private practice these costs may be passed on to the patient, the ability to do so under other national systems of pay may be restricted. In obtaining consent from the patients these differences may be relevant and consideration should be given to discussing these with the patient.

In Chapter 3, the importance of setting out all the treatment options to the patient once a diagnosis has been made was described. A definitive diagnosis is not always clear. Advising the patient of probable diagnosis, treatments options and other important issues such as costs (where relevant), complications, and limitations are essential to allow the patient to make the right decision for themselves. Before embarking on endodontic treatment the patient should be informed about:

- How the treatment will be carried out;
- How long it will take (expected duration and number of appointments);
- Post-operative discomfort/pain and how to manage this;
- Information about returning if problems occur (e.g. pain, swelling);
- Requirements for further treatment (e.g. crowns, posts, cuspal coverage);
- Costs of endodontic treatment and any recommended further treatment.

Providing this information enables the patients to consider whether they would like to undertake the procedure, and may alert the clinician to issues such as an upcoming holiday or important engagements which may delay the treatment plan. Much of this information will be provided verbally, with the patient encouraged to ask questions to ensure they understand what has been said. It is useful to support this verbal discussion with written information, such as patient information leaflets and a consent form. It should be stressed that a signed consent form is not a panacea. Consent forms serve only to confirm the quantity, not the quality, of information provided to the patient.

How should inadequate root canal fillings be prevented or managed?

The largest source of complaints and claims in endodontics arise from the technical failure to adequately fill the root canal system in the presence of persistent infection. This may include: missed root canals (Fig. 10.2a); overextended (Fig. 10.2b), underextended (Fig. 10.2c), and/or poorly compacted root canal fillings (Fig. 10.2d); the use of unacceptable root canal filling materials, e.g. silver points (Fig. 10.2e) or formaldehyde pastes. A technically inadequate root canal filling can be indicative of inadequate root canal preparation, i.e. the root canal system has not been adequately disinfected.

The judicious use of radiographs is an important part of reducing the risk of inadequate root canal filling. Many clinicians use electronic apex locators (EALs) to assess the working length of root canals and avoid taking radiographs during treatment. It is still important to take intraoperative radiograph(s) (e.g. a working length and/or master point radiograph). Post-operative radiographs should always be taken to confirm the quality of the root canal filling. If there are radiographic shortcomings with the quality of the root canal filling, this would then be an opportunity to outline these to the patients with options on how to manage them.

There are situations when a patient sees another clinician (e.g. an emergency dentist) after completion of endodontic treatment. Clinicians should be sensitive when describing the quality of a root canal filling which has been carried out by a colleague. Any inadequacies should be described diplomatically and using objective rather than subjective descriptions. This should be in the context of the nature of the endodontic condition/disease (e.g. infection is the essential cause of periapical periodontitis and not necessarily an overextended root canal filling), the complexity of the anatomy of the root canal system, and the intricacies of the endodontic procedure. A significant number of complaints are generated when another clinician makes injudicious comments without knowing the full details of treatment provided elsewhere.

How should separated instruments be prevented or managed?

It is not negligent to separate an instrument in a root canal if the instruments are used in a reasonable manner, such as running the correct speed for machine-driven instruments and using the instrument in accordance with the manufacturer's instructions. However, if it does occur (Fig. 10.3) the patient *must* be informed and advised about the options which will include extraction of the tooth, completing root

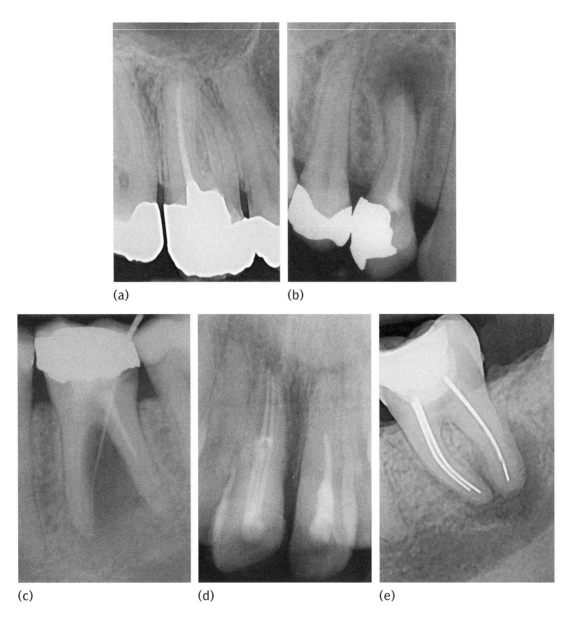

(a)   (b)

(c)   (d)   (e)

Figure 10.2 Root canal fillings with inadequate technical quality: (a) no root canal filling in the mesio-buccal root canal of a maxillary molar tooth; (b) overextended root canal filling associated with a maxillary premolar tooth; (c) underextended root canal fillings associated with a mandibular molar tooth; (d) poorly compacted root canal filling associated with a maxillary incisor tooth; (e) silver point root canal fillings associated with a mandibular molar tooth.

canal treatment with the instrument retained *in situ*, or arranging referral to a specialist in endodontics. It is important that this advice is recorded in the clinical records. Research indicates that the retention of a separated instrument in an adequately disinfected root canal system will not significantly alter the outcome of endodontic treatment. The following guidance will help to reduce the risk of a separated instrument:

- Use the instrument in accordance with the manufacturer's instructions;

- Single-visit use of instruments to reduce the risk of fracture due to cyclical fatigue;

- Avoid using NiTi files in root canals with sharp curvatures;

- Avoid forcing an instrument into a narrow or partially calcified root canal;

- Check the instrument before and after use for any deformation;

- Immediately discard any deformed instrument;

- Measure the instrument before and after use.

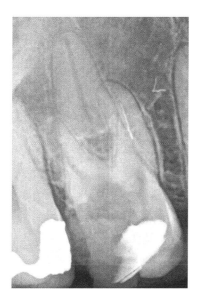

Figure 10.3 Separated file in the mesial-buccal root of a maxillary molar tooth.

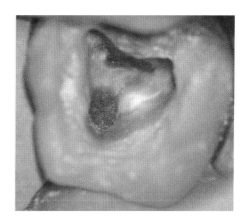

Figure 10.4 Perforation of the pulp chamber wall of a maxillary molar tooth. This occurred when the clinician was attempting to locate the entrance to the disto-buccal root canal.

How should perforations be prevented or managed?

Perforations may occur in any part of the root canal system. Examples include, perforation of the pulp chamber wall or floor when attempting to locate the entrance to a root canal (Fig. 10.4), or strip perforation of the root canal wall when carrying out mechanical preparation or post preparation (Fig. 10.5a,b). If a perforation occurs, the patient *must* be informed and advised about the options which will include extraction of the tooth, repair of the perforation, or arranging for its management by referral to a specialist in endodontics. This advice should be recorded in the clinical notes. The following guidance will help to reduce the risk of perforation:

- Use a preoperative radiograph to estimate the depth of the pulp chamber floor and the angulation of the root(s).

- Consider creating the access cavity prior to placement of rubber dam as the rubber dam may mask the angulation of the root(s).
- Consider removing the entire coronal restoration to aid vision and location of root canals.
- Use a bur with a non-cutting, safe-ended tip after initial access has been made into the pulp chamber.
- Precurve stainless steel files, especially stiffer files of ISO size >20.
- Avoid aggressive linear filing of the root canal wall closest to the furcation region. Aggressive use of Gates Glidden drills should also be avoided.

What risks are associated with using sodium hypochlorite as an irrigant?

Sodium hypochlorite (NaOCl) is the irrigant of choice and whilst 0.5 per cent concentration is effective, many clinicians use undiluted commercially available household bleach at concentrations of up to 5 per cent. This raises two issues relating to safety and the appropriateness of using a household product that is not licensed for medical/dental use.

Sodium hypochlorite, especially at higher concentrations, has the ability to dissolve organic tissue and this is favourable for dissolving pulp tissue remnants in the root canal. However, extrusion of NaOCl into the periapical tissues can cause significant damage to the surrounding tissues (Fig. 10.6), including neurological damage, and in some cases this can be life-threatening. Caution must be exercised when using higher concentrations of NaOCl and precautions must be taken to prevent extrusion through the apex of a tooth or iatrogenic perforations. The number of reported cases of

adverse incidents with NaOCl has increased over the past 10 years (Fig. 10.7). The following guidance will help to reduce the risk of an adverse incident:

- Provide patients with eye shields/goggles and bibs to protect from spillages;
- Use rubber dam;
- Follow the above guidance for reducing the risk of perforation;
- Determine the working length using an accurate method;
- Use a side-venting needle that has been premeasured to the working length;
- Use a syringe with threads (Luer-Lok) so the needle can be securely screwed on;

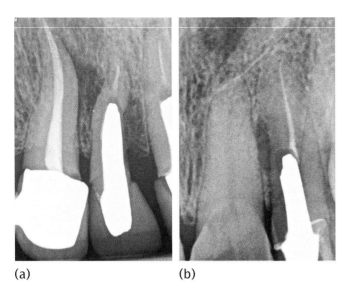

(a)   (b)

Figure 10.5 (a,b) Post perforations and lateral radiolucencies associated with maxillary incisor teeth.

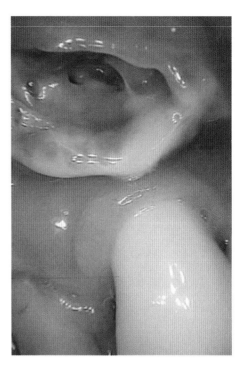

Figure 10.6 Ulcerated intraoral soft tissues following a sodium hypochlorite (NaOCl) accident.

Courtesy of Dr Steve Williams. Adapted from Patel S and Duncan H (2011) *Pitt Ford's Problem-Based Learning in Endodontology*. Printed with permission from Wiley-Blackwell.

- Do not force or bind the needle in the root canal;
- Use gentle finger (not thumb) pressure to introduce the irrigant into the root canal.

Some clinicians may say that they have used household bleach for irrigation in endodontic treatment for many years without adverse effects. It should be remembered that household bleach is marketed for stain removal in fabrics and disinfection of domestic surfaces. There are commercially available NaOCl solutions that are licensed for intraoral use and it may be more appropriate to use these in endodontics.

Patients may report an allergy/hypersensitivity to chlorine. Ideally, this should be confirmed by allergy testing. It would be advisable not to use NaOCl during endodontic treatment in these patients. There are alternatives irrigants, such as chlorhexidine gluconate and iodine potassium iodide; however, these are not as effective as NaOCl. The patient should be informed of this and the possible effect on the outcome of endodontic treatment.

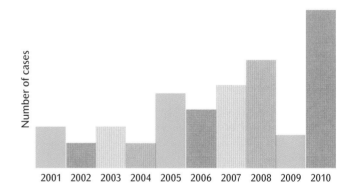

Figure 10.7 Number of reported cases of adverse incidents with sodium hypochlorite (NaOCl) between 2001 and 2010.

Why should rubber dam be used?

Rubber dam has many advantages which benefit both the patient and the clinician. Unfortunately, several survey studies have reported that the use of rubber dam by clinicians is low. From a dento-legal perspective, the purpose of rubber dam is to protect the oropharynx. This may be protection from instruments (e.g. files) or caustic substances (e.g. NaOCl) being swallowed or inhaled. The use of rotary instrumentation is increasingly more common so these handpiece retained instruments are no more likely to be swallowed or inhaled than handpiece retained burs. There are other methods of preventing instruments slipping and being accidentally dropped into the patient's mouth, such as parachute chains and tying a length of dental floss through the handle of the endodontic file and retaining the end of it. In the absence of these safety devices, if a patient were to swallow or inhale an instrument, the chances of defending any legal claim arising out of the incident would be limited.

Fractured teeth

Restoration of the endodontically treated tooth is discussed in Chapter 7. It is generally recommended that endodontically treated molars be restored with a cast restoration that provides cuspal protection (e.g. crown, onlay). Endodontically treated molars are considered more susceptible to fracturing compared with their vital counterparts, especially if the tooth has little remaining tooth structure and the patient has a parafunctional habit. Studies have shown that these teeth will survive longer with a cast restoration that provides cuspal protection. It is usually recommended that a patient proceed with cuspal protection within a few weeks after endodontic treatment, subject to the tooth being symptom-free. Some patients may want to delay cuspal protection until the outcome of endodontic treatment is deemed favourable. These patients should be informed that outcome is usually assessed at least one year after completion of endodontic treatment and there is a risk that the tooth may fracture while waiting (Fig. 10.8). Patients' should be advised of cuspal protection from the outset and this should be recorded in the clinical records.

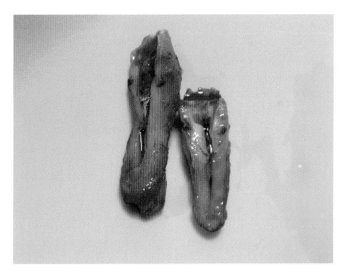

Figure 10.8 Extracted endodontically treated premolar tooth which had a complete vertical tooth and root fracture.

Record keeping

The quality and standard of record keeping is usually very high amongst undergraduate dental students and recently qualified dentists. Over time, however, the detail recorded diminishes with the most often quoted reason being lack time.

Most endodontic procedures in general practice start with the patient attending complaining of pain and/or swelling. A detailed examination of the patient is necessary as outlined in Chapter 3. Pertinent details should be recorded, e.g. type of pain, duration, exacerbating and relieving factors, as well as results of special tests. It is also essential to record the discussion of the various treatment options. Many practices are now computerized and custom screens with prompts to ask the right questions are readily available.

These details often make the difference in a complaint or clinical negligence claim which may be made many months or even years after the event. The question 'Why was endodontic treatment necessary for this patient?' may well be asked. You will have only your notes and records to rely on to establish not only why, but also what was treated, when it was treated, how it was treated, and what further treatment was recommended. Remember: *if it was not written down, it did not happen.* Courts are more likely to rely on the evidence of a patient since they usually have one dentist. Clinicians will have many patients and are unlikely to remember in any great detail what happened on a particular appointment without the prompting of contemporaneous records.

Conclusion

Learning from your mistakes is the hallmark of a professional. Reflecting on what has gone wrong and how it can be improved makes the difference between delivering better healthcare outcomes and making the same mistake again. Of course, nobody welcomes complaints in whatever form they come to you. It is a challenge to your professional integrity and can be quite dispiriting and stressful, particularly when you feel you have tried your best. Beneath every complaint, no matter how unjustified it first appears, there is something to learn. Even when things go drastically wrong (e.g. the patient swallows an instrument, or a file separates in the root canal), it is how the situation is managed that will make the difference.

The world of endodontics will continue to change with a plethora of gadgets, new concepts, and new techniques. Clinicians need to ensure what they do is as evidence based as possible, and new materials and techniques are used with caution until their efficacy has been established. When endodontic treatment is carried out well, it is rewarding to the clinician, but more importantly allows the patient to obtain more function and appearance that may not have been possible otherwise.

Summary points

- Valid consent is a continuing process that involves the patient being competent, giving voluntary permission, and being given information on which to make their decision.

- When giving a patient information, this should include the probable diagnosis, treatment options, and other important issues such as costs, complications, and limitations.

- In primary dental care in the UK, endodontics has the highest number of legal claims in comparison with other dental treatments. Most complaints and claims arise from an inadequate root canal filling in the presence of residual infection and separated instruments.

- It is important to recognize when something goes wrong and how to manage the situation. This will start with good communication with the patient and detailed record keeping. Management may include referral to a specialist.

Suggested further reading

Bolitho v. *City and Hackney Health Authority* [1997] UKHL 46; [1998] AC 232; [1997] 4 All ER 771; [1997] 3 WLR 1151.

Bowden JR, Ethuandan M and Brennan PA (2006) Life threatening airway obstruction secondary to hypochlorite extrusion during root canal treatment. *Oral Surgery, Oral Medicine, Oral Pathology, Oral Radiology, and Endodontology* **101**, 402–4.

Chaudhry H, Wildan TM, Popat S, Anand R and Dhariwal D (2011) Before you reach for the bleach. *British Dental Journal* **210**, 157–60.

D'Cruz L (2008) The successful management of complaints—turning threats into opportunities. *Dental Update* **35**, 182–6.

Dental Protection Ltd (2009) *Risk Management Module 2 – Endodontics*. London, UK: DPL Publications.

Ng YL, Mann V and Gulabivala K (2010) Tooth survival following non-surgical root canal treatment: a systematic review of the literature. *International Endodontic Journal* **43**, 171–89.

Salehrabi R and Rotstein I (2004) Endodontic treatment outcomes in a large patient population in the USA: an epidemiological study. *Journal of Endodontics* **30**, 846–50.

Sidaway v. *Board of Governors of the Bethlem Royal Hospital* [1985] AC871.

Webber J (2010) Risk management in clinical practice. Part 4. Endodontics. *British Dental Journal* **209**, 161–70.

Online Resource Centre

To help you to develop and apply your knowledge and skills further, we have provided interactive learning resources online at http://www.oxfordtextbooks.co.uk/orc/patel/

Index

Page numbers in *italics* represent figures, those in **bold** represent tables.